INTERMITTENT FASTING
FOR WOMEN
OVER 50

**Detoxify, Regenerate, and Challenge Aging a Secret
Metabolic Boost to Lose Weight.
Get Fit Feel 30 Again
with 120 Recipes and a 28-Day Meal Plan**

Laure Leller

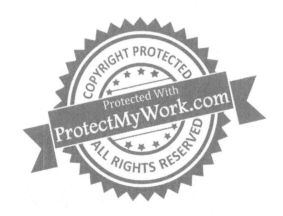

Table of Contents

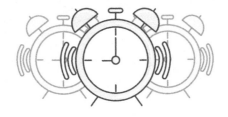

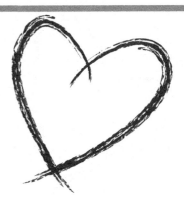

Table of Contents

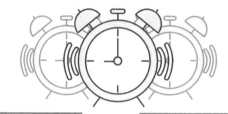

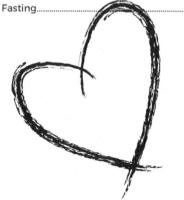

This book was written to promote awareness of the importance of paying attention to what one eats and to offer the possibility to vary one's cuisine. However, it is not meant to be a replacement for medical advice.

By responding to frequently asked concerns, offering solutions, and offering guidance, it is intended that people can gain a better understanding of eating disorders and what can lead to inadequate nutrition.

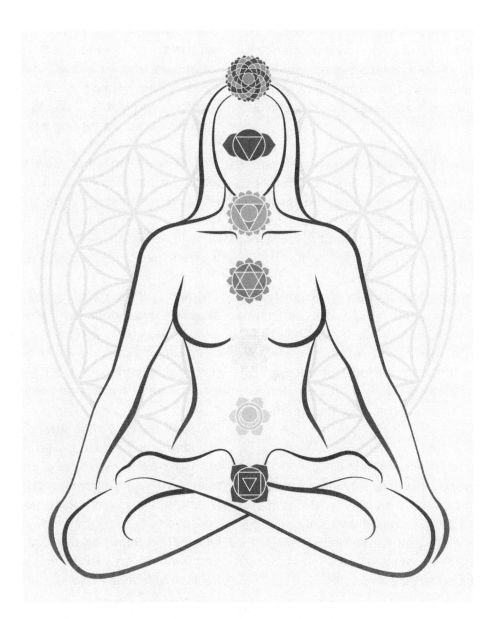

Introduction

Intermittent fasting has emerged as a widespread eating practice with significant benefits for people approaching age 50 and beyond. Unlike traditional diets focusing on specific food choices, intermittent fasting focuses on when to eat, presenting a unique and intriguing approach to overall health and well-being.

Throughout human evolution, periodic starvation has been a natural phenomenon, as ancient populations did not have access to supermarkets or refrigerators year-round. This led our bodies to adapt to function efficiently for long periods without food. Intermittent fasting takes advantage of this inherent ability, making it a natural and instinctive eating pattern for our bodies.

The main goal of intermittent fasting is not to limit the types of foods consumed but rather to create distinct periods of eating and fasting. In this way, our bodies undergo several physiological changes that can lead to numerous health benefits.

One of the main benefits of intermittent fasting is its ability to facilitate weight loss. By limiting the food window, individuals tend to consume fewer calories, reducing overall caloric intake naturally. In addition, periods of fasting can cause the body to draw on stored fat reserves as an energy source, promoting fat burning and weight loss.

In addition, intermittent fasting can have a positive impact on metabolism. Regular fasting helps optimize insulin sensitivity, promoting a healthier metabolic rate and better blood sugar utilization. This can be especially beneficial for older women, as it boosts a healthy metabolism and better blood sugar control.

Another fascinating aspect of intermittent fasting is its influence on hormonal health. By promoting efficient insulin sensitivity and blood sugar regulation, this eating pattern can impact essential hormones such as leptin and ghrelin, which play a crucial role in appetite management and calorie balance. For women who struggle with stubborn fat despite following a healthy diet and exercise program, intermittent fasting can be a valuable tool to promote fat loss.

Intermittent fasting is not a one-size-fits-all approach; it is crucial to approach it with awareness and individual health conditions in mind. Older women or those with specific medical problems should consult their physician before adopting a fasting regimen.

It is essential to emphasize that intermittent fasting is not simply about skipping meals or drastically reducing caloric intake. On the contrary, it encourages a holistic lifestyle change involving healthier food choices and maintaining adequate portions.

To begin intermittent fasting, individuals can choose from various fasting methods, such as every-other-day fasting or time-restricted daily eating. Some may fast for specific hours daily, while others may choose fasting days interspersed with non-fasting days.

By embracing intermittent fasting in a thoughtful and individualized way, women over 50 can experience improvements in weight management, hormonal balance, and overall health. This comprehensive and exciting approach goes beyond the repetitive information found on the web, offering a fresh perspective on achieving wellness and a balanced lifestyle in old age.

CHAPTER I

Unlocking the Power of Intermittent Fasting

1.1: Redefining Fasting – An Evolutionary Approach to Health

Fasting, defined as abstaining from eating anything, has been ingrained in human history, shaped by our ancestors' need to adapt to periods of feast and famine. However, the modern approach to fasting has evolved significantly, leading to the emergence of intermittent fasting as a revolutionary nutritional strategy.

Intermittent fasting involves adopting specific fasting intervals over a few days, alternating with periods of food consumption, providing freedom and flexibility in its implementation. Unlike traditional diets that dictate strict food choices, intermittent fasting prioritizes the timing of eating and fasting windows, allowing the body to access its natural healing mechanisms.

Drawing inspiration from our ancestral past, where food scarcity was common, intermittent fasting taps into the body's innate ability to function optimally during fasting periods. The deliberate action of depriving the body of food for more than six hours triggers metabolic changes that promote overall well-being, such as cellular repair, autophagy, and hormone regulation.

1.2: Intermittent Fasting Unveiled – A Revolutionary Nutritional Strategy

Intermittent fasting stands apart from conventional diets and eating patterns by focusing on when food is consumed rather than specific food restrictions. It offers a range of methods to create fasting intervals, allowing individuals to customize their approach according to their goals and lifestyle.

One of the most common methods is the 16/8 approach, where individuals fast for 16 hours and have an 8-hour eating window. Another form involves cyclic fasting to reduce overall daily caloric intake. Intermittent fasting's main objective is to divert the body's attention from constant food digestion, enabling it to experience metabolic changes that lead to benefits like weight loss and improved body composition.

Scientific research supports intermittent fasting's positive impact on metabolism, insulin resistance, inflammation, and various health markers. It promotes metabolic flexibility, allowing the body to switch between glucose and ketones as energy sources. This shift to ketosis, where fat becomes the primary fuel source, aids fat-burning and cellular rejuvenation.

1.3: Embracing Freedom – The Flexibility and Customization of Intermittent Fasting

Intermittent fasting provides a liberating sense of flexibility compared to rigid diet plans. It allows individuals to tailor their fasting schedule to their preferences, body type, and nutritional needs. The primary goal remains to achieve a better metabolism, healthy body weight, and an active lifestyle.

During the eating window, individuals can consume a wide range of foods, focusing on low-calorie, nutrient-dense options such as meat, fish, eggs, whole grains, legumes, and fresh fruits. Minimizing simple sugars and choosing low glycemic index foods helps maintain stable energy levels.

Intermittent fasting comprises various methods of food abstinence, including alternate-day fasting, daily restrictions, and periodic fasting. While the approach may differ, the ultimate goal remains consistent—unlocking the body's self-healing mechanisms by diverting energy from constant digestion.

The positive effects of intermittent fasting extend beyond physical health. It fosters self-discipline, aids in overcoming bad eating habits, and enhances mental clarity. The practice promotes the production of beta-hydroxybutyrate (BHB), a substance that can combat chronic inflammation and offers potential benefits in managing inflammatory-based diseases.

The working principle of intermittent fasting revolves around utilizing stored energy, such as body fat, during fasting periods. The body shifts from a state of absorption to a form of fasting, leading to fat-burning and activating restorative processes. Several health advantages of intermittent fasting include less inflammation, improved cardiovascular health, and increased cognitive function. Intermittent fasting also influences insulin levels, human growth hormones, cellular repair, and gene expression.

Individuals can choose from various intermittent fasting methods, such as the 16/8 approach, alternate-day fasting, or occasional fasting. Despite the numerous benefits, it is essential to approach intermittent fasting with consideration for individual factors, and women may require a modified approach due to the impact on hormone regulation.

The science behind intermittent fasting is rooted in the body's natural ability to switch between states of absorption and fasting. When fasting, the body taps into stored energy reserves, leading to fat utilization and a range of beneficial effects on metabolic health.

To embark on an intermittent fasting journey, individuals can start with short fasting periods and gradually increase their fasting window. Proper hydration is essential during fasting periods, and it's crucial to engage in physical activity in a way that complements the fasting schedule.

By embracing intermittent fasting as a lifestyle choice, individuals can unlock the power of their body's self-healing and restorative capabilities, promoting longevity, vitality, and overall well-being. The potential benefits of intermittent fasting are vast and extend to physical and mental health, offering a promising approach to optimal living in the modern world.

CHAPTER II

Unveiling the Various Methods of Intermittent Fasting - A Comprehensive Overview

Intermittent fasting offers a range of methods to accommodate individual preferences, lifestyles, and health goals. Understanding the various fasting protocols is crucial to finding the most suitable approach.

The choice of method should be based on personal preferences, lifestyle, and health considerations. It is essential to start gradually and listen to the body's cues to ensure a safe and sustainable intermittent fasting journey. As usual, speaking with a healthcare provider before starting an intermittent fast is advised, especially for people with specific health issues or medical problems.

2.1: The 16/8 Method - Time-Restricted Eating for Beginners

The 16/8 method is one of the most popular and beginner-friendly approaches to intermittent fasting. It entails cutting the eating window to only eight hours daily and observing a 16-hour fast. Time-restricted eating is another name for this strategy.

How to Follow the 16/8 Method:

You can choose your fasting window: Decide on a suitable fasting period from 8 PM to 12 PM the next day, allowing an 8-hour eating window from 12 PM to 8 PM.

Stay hydrated: During the fasting period, drink plenty of water, herbal teas, or black coffee without added sugar or cream to stay hydrated and suppress hunger.

Balanced meals: Ensure that your meals during the eating window balance nutrients, including proteins, healthy fats, and whole grains, to meet your body's needs.

Benefits and Considerations:

The 16/8 method is relatively easy to adapt to daily life as it does not require significant changes in meal patterns. It aids in weight loss by reducing overall caloric intake and improves insulin sensitivity. However, it is essential to prioritize the quality of food consumed during the eating window to maximize the health benefits of this method.

2.2: Alternate-Day Fasting – Challenging but Rewarding

Fasting days and eating days are alternated during alternate-day fasting. On days when you fast, you consume much fewer calories than you would on a regular eating day.

How to Follow Alternate-Day Fasting:

Choose fasting days: Decide the number of fasting days per week, typically 1-3 days.

Calorie restriction on fasting days: On fasting days, consume only 500-600 calories to promote fat burning while still providing essential nutrients.

Adequate hydration: Drink water daily to keep your body hydrated when fasting.

Benefits and Considerations:

Alternate-day fasting has shown promise in promoting weight loss, improving cardiovascular health, and enhancing metabolic function. However, adhering to the strict calorie restriction on fasting days may be challenging for some individuals. It is crucial to consult a healthcare professional before attempting this method, especially for those with underlying health conditions.

2.3: The 5:2 Diet – Balanced Eating with Periodic Fasting

The 5:2 diet is a well-known kind of intermittent fasting that calls for regular eating five days a week and calorie restriction on two days that are not consecutive.

How to Follow the 5:2 Diet:

Select fasting days: Choose two non-consecutive days in a week for fasting; a typical eating day should come between each.

Limitations on calories on fasting days: On days when you fast, keep your calorie intake to 500–600 calories and focus on nutrient-dense meals.

Balanced eating regularly: Consume a balanced diet on the remaining five days to meet nutritional needs.

Benefits and Considerations:

The 5:2 diet offers a balanced approach to intermittent fasting, allowing individuals to enjoy regular meals most of the week while still experiencing the benefits of fasting on specific days. It aids in weight loss, improves insulin sensitivity, and may positively affect brain health. However, some individuals may find calorie restriction challenging on fasting days.

2.4: The Eat-Stop-Eat Method – Occasional 24-Hour Fasting

The Eat-Stop-Eat approach calls for fasting once or twice weekly for 24 hours. This approach requires more extended periods of fasting but is performed on only some days.

How to Follow the Eat-Stop-Eat Method:

Choose fasting days: Select one or two non-consecutive days per week for fasting.
Fasting duration: Fast for 24 hours, from dinner to dinner or breakfast to breakfast, depending on personal preference.

Stay hydrated: Consume water, herbal teas, or black coffee during fasting.

Benefits and Considerations:
The Eat-Stop-Eat method offers the benefits of more extended fasting periods, promoting greater fat-burning and metabolic improvements. It may aid in weight loss and support cellular repair processes. However, the longer fasting duration may not be suitable for everyone, and individuals with specific health concerns should consult a healthcare professional before attempting this method.

2.5: The Warrior Diet – Undereating During the Day, Feast at Nigh

The Warrior Diet follows a unique approach: individuals undereat or fast during the day and consume one large meal at night.

How to Follow the Warrior Diet:

Undereating during the day: Consume small portions of raw fruits, vegetables, and light protein sources.

Feast at night: Have a single, substantial meal that balances proteins, good fats, and carbs.

Benefits and Considerations:
The Warrior Diet is inspired by ancient warrior cultures, where a substantial meal at night followed limited food availability during the day. This approach allows for greater metabolic flexibility and provides an opportunity for self-control during the day. It might only be suited for some, though, as some people could find it difficult to eat too little during the day and a big meal at night.

2.6: The OMAD (One Meal a Day) – Minimalist Fasting Approach

The OMAD (One Meal a Day) approach involves fasting for 23 hours and eating all daily calories in one large meal.

How to Follow the OMAD Method:

One meal a day: Consume all daily calories in one meal, typically at the same time each day.
Nutrient-dense meal: Ensure that the meal includes a variety of nutrients, proteins, healthy fats, and fiber-rich foods.

Benefits and Considerations:
OMAD is a minimalist fasting approach that simplifies meal planning and timing. It can lead to significant calorie reduction and weight loss while providing a sense of food freedom during the eating window. However, it may be challenging for some individuals to meet their nutritional needs in one meal, and it may not be suitable for those with specific dietary requirements or medical conditions.

2.7: Customizing Intermittent Fasting – Finding What Works for You

The beauty of intermittent fasting lies in its flexibility and customizability. Different methods suit individuals based on lifestyle, health goals, and personal preferences. Some may prefer shorter fasting periods with daily restrictions, while others may find longer fasting intervals or alternate-day fasting more suitable.

Key Considerations for Customizing Intermittent Fasting:

Individual needs: Consider personal health conditions, daily routines, and physical activity levels when choosing intermittent fasting.

Gradual approach: Start with a milder method, such as the 16/8 approach, and gradually transition to more extended fasting periods if desired.
Nutrient-dense eating: Regardless of the method chosen, prioritize nutrient-dense foods to support overall health during eating windows.

Benefits and Considerations:
Customizing intermittent fasting allows individuals to find a sustainable approach that fits seamlessly into their lifestyle. It can improve metabolic health and weight loss and enhance overall well-being. However, it is essential to be mindful of individual needs and consult a healthcare professional, especially those with existing health conditions or specific dietary requirements.

2.8: Tips for a Successful Intermittent Fasting Journey

Embarking on an intermittent fasting journey can be a transformative and empowering experience. To ensure success and make the most of this dietary approach, consider the following tips:

Start Gradually

If you are new to intermittent fasting, begin with a more manageable method, such as the 16/8 approach. Allow your body to adapt slowly to the fasting periods and gradually extend fasting durations if desired.

Stay Hydrated

During fasting periods, focus on hydrating with water, herbal teas, and black coffee. Proper hydration not only helps suppress hunger but also supports overall well-being.

Prioritize Nutrient-Dense Foods

Choose nutritious, well-balanced meals when breaking your fast. To achieve your nutritional needs, emphasize lean proteins, healthy fats, whole grains, and fruits and vegetables.

Take Note of Your Body

Pay attention to your body's cues and modify your fasting strategy. If a particular approach is causing discomfort or not aligning with your lifestyle, explore alternative methods that better suit your needs.

Be Mindful of Exercise

Moderate exercise can complement intermittent fasting and enhance its benefits. However, intense workouts during fasting periods may be challenging. Consider scheduling exercise during eating windows for optimal performance and recovery.

Plan Ahead

Plan your meals and fasting periods ahead of time to avoid impulsive and unhealthy food choices. A well-thought-out meal plan can help you stay on track and achieve your health goals.

Look for accountability and support

Consider joining a community or finding a fasting buddy to share experiences and provide mutual support. Having someone to discuss challenges and successes with can make your intermittent fasting journey more enjoyable and sustainable.

2.9: Intermittent Fasting and Exercise – A Winning Combination

Integrating intermittent fasting with exercise can be a powerful combination for overall health and well-being. When approached mindfully, training can enhance the benefits of intermittent fasting and vice versa.

Pre-Workout Considerations: If you prefer to exercise during fasting periods, focus on low to moderate-intensity activities such as walking, yoga, or light strength training. These exercises can be sustainable during fasting and help burn stored fat effectively.

Post-Workout Nutrition: After a workout, prioritize refueling your body with a balanced meal rich in protein, carbohydrates, and healthy fats. This helps replenish glycogen stores and supports muscle recovery.

Monitor your body's reaction to exercise when you're fasting by closely monitoring it.
If you experience excessive fatigue, dizziness, or other discomforts, consider adjusting your workout schedule to align better with your eating windows.

Hydration Matters: Staying hydrated during exercise is crucial, especially during fasting. Drink plenty of water to maintain optimal performance and prevent dehydration.

2.10: Addressing Concerns and Potential Risks

While intermittent fasting has shown promising results for many individuals, it may only suit some. Addressing potential concerns and risks can help ensure a safe and successful fitful fasting journey.

Underlying Health Conditions: Before beginning intermittent fasting, speak with a medical expert if you have any health issues or concerns. A modified strategy or strict monitoring may be necessary for diseases like diabetes or eating disorders.

Nutritional Adequacy: Ensure that your eating windows provide sufficient nutrients to support your body's needs. Nutrient-dense foods should be a priority to avoid deficiencies and promote overall well-being.

Pregnancy and Lactation: Intermittent fasting is generally not recommended for pregnant or breastfeeding individuals, as it may not nourish the mother and the developing baby.

Mindful Eating: Avoid overcompensating with unhealthy food choices during eating windows. Intermittent fasting is not a license to indulge in excessively unhealthy foods, as this can undermine the benefits of fasting.

CONSIDERATIONS

A flexible and successful strategy for improving health and well-being is intermittent fasting. People can choose a fasting strategy that fits their demands and lifestyles because of its various approaches. Intermittent fasting has some advantages, including better metabolism, higher energy, and improved mental clarity, when accompanied by a balanced diet, exercise, and a mindful attitude.

As with any dietary or lifestyle change, listening to your body, seeking professional guidance when needed, and making sustainable choices is essential. The journey of intermittent fasting is not about deprivation or strict rules; instead, it is a path toward a healthier and more fulfilling life. Embrace the power of intermittent fasting, and unlock its potential to elevate your mind, body, and spirit to new heights.

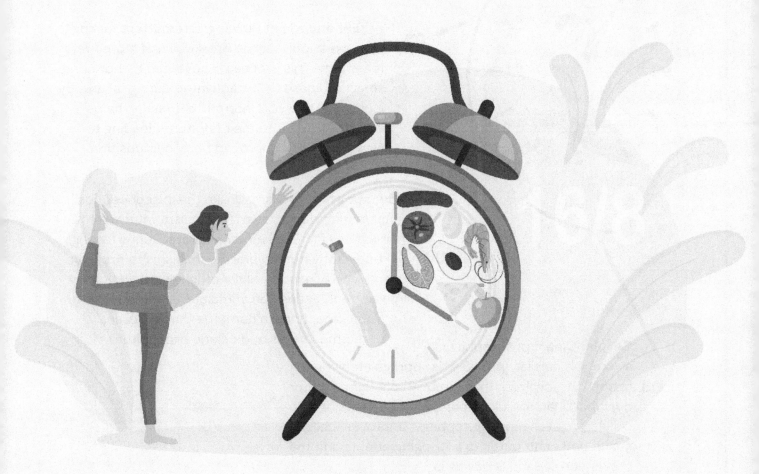

CHAPTER III

The Fascinating Science Behind Intermittent Fasting

3.1: Metabolic Magic – How Intermittent Fasting Ignites the Body's Potential

Intermittent fasting's profound impact on metabolism lies at the heart of its effectiveness as a dietary approach. The body goes through several metabolic changes that improve functioning and foster health advantages during fasting.

01 Energy Utilization: When fasting, the body switches from utilizing glucose as its primary energy source to relying on stored fats. Insulin secretion falls when blood glucose levels rise, allowing fat cells to release stored fatty acids. These fatty acids are then broken down into ketones, which become the body's alternative fuel source.

02 Enhanced Fat Burning: Intermittent fasting promotes lipolysis, the breakdown of stored fats for energy. This process is governed by hormone-sensitive lipase (HSL), activated during fasting. By increasing lipolysis, intermittent fasting helps individuals tap into their fat stores, leading to weight loss and improved body composition.

03 Boosting Metabolism: Unlike the misconception that fasting slows down metabolism, intermittent fasting may increase metabolic rate. During fasting, the body activates several mechanisms to preserve energy and enhance cellular efficiency. Additionally, intermittent fasting can stimulate the production of norepinephrine, a hormone that increases thermogenesis and calorie expenditure.

04 Cellular Cleanup: Autophagy, a crucial cellular process is upregulated during fasting. It involves the removal of damaged or dysfunctional cellular components, leading to cellular rejuvenation. Autophagy improves cellular health and contributes to anti-aging effects and the prevention of various diseases.

3.2: Rewriting the Genetic Code – Cellular Repair and Anti–Aging Benefits

Intermittent fasting goes beyond its impact on metabolism; it also influences gene expression and cellular repair mechanisms, contributing to anti-aging benefits and improved cellular health.

Gene Expression: Fasting triggers changes in gene expression, influencing the activity of various genes related to longevity, cellular repair, and stress resistance. Activating longevity genes, such as SIRT1 and anti-inflammatory genes, can enhance cellular resilience and extend lifespan.

Anti-Aging Effects: By promoting autophagy and eliminating damaged cellular components, intermittent fasting contributes to anti-aging effects. By clearing out dysfunctional proteins and organelles, cells can function optimally, leading to improved tissue health and overall longevity.

Oxidative Stress and Antioxidant Defense: Intermittent fasting helps balance oxidative stress, reducing excessive free radical production. During fasting, the body experiences a temporary increase in oxidative stress, which acts as a hormetic response, prompting it to upregulate its antioxidant defense mechanisms. This adaptive response strengthens the body's ability to combat oxidative damage.

Longevity Pathways: The mTOR and IGF-1 signaling pathways, as well as other pathways involved in aging, are all activated by intermittent fasting. These pathways are essential for controlling cellular metabolism, aging, and growth. By modulating these pathways, intermittent fasting may support healthy aging and longevity.

3.3: Hormonal Symphony – Insulin, Growth Hormones, and Optimal Fat Burning

The body's reaction to fasting periods and the advantages that follow for fat-burning and metabolic health are greatly influenced by the complex interactions of hormones that occur during intermittent fasting.

Insulin Sensitivity: The term "insulin sensitivity" describes how receptive the body is to the hormone insulin, which controls blood sugar levels. By improving insulin sensitivity, intermittent fasting can lower the chance of developing insulin resistance and type 2 diabetes. Increased insulin sensitivity also facilitates fat burning by enhancing glucose intake.

Growth Hormones: It has been demonstrated that intermittent fasting increases the synthesis of growth hormones like human growth hormone (HGH). Growth hormones are vital in tissue repair, muscle growth, and overall metabolism. Higher levels of growth hormones during fasting periods can accelerate fat burning and preserve lean muscle mass.

Glucagon and Glycogen: The hormone glucagon is produced when fasting, causing the liver's glycogen (stored glucose) to break down more quickly. Once glycogen reserves are exhausted, the body switches to alternate fuel sources, such as lipids. This procedure promotes fat burning and aids in the maintenance of steady blood glucose levels.

Leptin and Ghrelin: Leptin and ghrelin are hormones that regulate hunger and satiety. Intermittent fasting can influence these hormones, reducing the need and better appetite control. Suppressing ghrelin, known as the hunger hormone, during fasting periods can help individuals adhere to their fasting schedule more easily.

CHAPTER IV

Embracing the Intermittent Fasting Lifestyle

4.1: Time-Restricted Feeding – Unveiling the 16/8, 24-hour, and Occasional Fasting

Intermittent fasting encompasses various approaches, each with its unique benefits and guidelines. A standard method of intermittent fasting is time-restricted feeding, which entails alternating between eating and fasting windows of time.

One standard time-restricted feeding method is the 16/8 protocol, where individuals fast for 16 hours and have an 8-hour eating window. This approach typically involves skipping breakfast and eating during midday and evening. Another variant is the 24-hour fasting method, where individuals fast for an entire day once or twice a week. This practice can be challenging for beginners but offers significant benefits when adopted correctly.

Occasional fasting is a more flexible approach, allowing individuals to choose specific days for fasting based on their schedule and preferences. Some might opt for one or two fasting days a week, while others fast intermittently throughout the month.

The Difference Between Methods:

The primary distinction between these methods lies in their fasting durations and frequency. While the 16/8 protocol involves fasting for 16 hours, the 24-hour fasting method includes extended fasting periods on specific days. On the other hand, occasional fasting allows for intermittent fasting periods dispersed throughout the week or month.

Choosing the Right Method:

The ideal intermittent fasting method depends on individual preferences, lifestyle, and health considerations. The 16/8 protocol is often favored by those seeking a consistent and manageable routine. It may suit individuals with regular daily schedules and those who prefer to fast daily but still enjoy regular meals within an 8-hour window.

The 24-hour fasting method is well-suited for individuals seeking more substantial health benefits and is willing to fast for extended periods on designated days. It requires more discipline and planning but can be highly effective for weight loss, cellular repair, and autophagy.

Occasional fasting provides flexibility, appealing to those who want to experience intermittent fasting benefits without strict adherence to a daily fasting schedule. This approach can be easily tailored to fit social events, special occasions, or any day when fasting might be more challenging.

Ultimately, the correct method depends on personal preferences, health goals, and consistently maintaining the fasting routine.

4.2: Customizing Your Journey – Finding the Perfect Fit for Your Lifestyle

One of the key strengths of intermittent fasting is its flexibility, allowing individuals to customize their fasting journey based on their unique needs and preferences. Here are some essential steps to help you find the perfect fit for your lifestyle:

Assess Your Goals: Determine what you want to achieve with intermittent fasting. Identifying your goals will guide your fasting approach, whether it's weight loss, improved metabolic health, increased energy, or better mental clarity.

Listen to Your Body: Take note of how it behaves to different fasting methods. Some individuals may find the 16/8 protocol more comfortable, while others may prefer occasional fasting for better adherence.

Start Slowly: If you're new to intermittent fasting, begin with a less restrictive approach, such as the 16/8 method. Gradually extend fasting durations or experiment with occasional fasting as you become more comfortable.

Be Mindful of Your Lifestyle: Consider your daily schedule, work commitments, social activities, and exercise routine when choosing a fasting method. Opt for an approach that complements your lifestyle rather than disrupting it.

Seek Professional Guidance: Before beginning intermittent fasting, speak with a healthcare provider or certified dietitian if you take medication, are pregnant, nursing, or have any pre-existing medical issues.

Stay Hydrated: Prioritize hydration during fasting times by consuming lots of water, herbal teas, or other calorie-free liquids to assist your body's processes.

Focus on Balanced Nutrition: Pick nutrient-dense, whole meals high in vitamins and minerals when you break your fast. Avoid compensating for fasting periods by overeating or consuming unhealthy foods.

Stay Consistent: To experience the full benefits of intermittent fasting, consistency is key. Establish a regular fasting routine that aligns with your goals and stick to it as much as possible.

4.3: Sustaining Success - Insights from the American Heart Association

The American Heart Association (AHA) has studied intermittent fasting and its potential impact on cardiovascular health and overall well-being. While intermittent fasting research is ongoing, the AHA's insights shed light on this dietary approach's potential benefits and considerations.

Cardio-Metabolic Benefits: Studies suggest intermittent fasting can improve several cardio-metabolic parameters, including blood pressure, blood glucose levels, insulin sensitivity, and lipid profiles. These advancements might lower the risk of type 2 diabetes and heart disease.

Weight Management: Intermittent fasting's effect on weight management is a significant area of interest. While individual results may vary, some individuals experience weight loss and better weight maintenance with intermittent fasting.

Reducing Inflammation: Chronic inflammation is a contributing factor to various chronic diseases. Some studies indicate that intermittent fasting helps reduce inflammation markers in the body, offering protective effects against inflammatory-based conditions.

Health and Longevity: Research on intermittent fasting's impact on lifespan and longevity pathways is still in its early stages. However, animal studies and some human trials have shown promising results, suggesting that intermittent fasting might extend lifespan and promote healthy aging.

It is crucial to remember that not everyone can benefit from intermittent fasting, particularly people with specific medical issues or dietary needs. Before beginning intermittent fasting, like any dietary modification, it is advised to speak with a healthcare provider, especially if you already have a medical condition, take medication, are pregnant, or are nursing. Incorporating intermittent fasting into a healthy and balanced lifestyle can yield positive results. Still, it is essential to approach it with mindfulness and care to ensure its long-term sustainability and benefits.

Additional Health Benefits:

Apart from heart health, diabetes management, and weight loss, intermittent fasting has shown promising effects on various other aspects of health:

Reduction of Inflammation: Chronic inflammation can result in weight gain and several health problems. Intermittent fasting has been found to reduce inflammation markers in some studies.

Psychological Well-being: Intermittent fasting has been linked to improved depression and compulsive eating behaviors while enhancing body image in obese adults.

Longer Life: Studies on animals suggest that intermittent fasting may extend lifespan, although the effects on humans are yet to be fully understood.

Preservation of Muscle Mass: Intermittent fasting appears more effective than constant calorie restriction in maintaining muscle mass, contributing to increased calorie burning even at rest.

Cognitive Effects: Intermittent fasting can enhance concentration and focus while boosting productivity.

Protection against Neuronal Degeneration: Intermittent fasting promotes autophagy, a cellular repair process that protects neurons and improves brain health.

Reduction of Insulin Levels and Insulin Resistance: Intermittent fasting increases insulin sensitivity, reducing the risk of insulin resistance and type 2 diabetes.

Reduced Risk of Chronic Diseases: Intermittent fasting may positively impact chronic autoimmune diseases and inhibit the growth of specific cancer cells.

Promotion of Immune Regulation: Intermittent fasting supports a healthy immune system by reducing inflammatory cytokines.

Ketosis: Intermittent fasting may lead to sporadic ketosis, in which the body utilizes energy from stored fat, promoting fat burning.

These various health benefits make intermittent fasting an enticing dietary approach for those seeking health improvements and disease prevention. It is essential to approach intermittent fasting with mindfulness, adopt a well-balanced diet, and consult a healthcare professional, particularly for individuals with specific health conditions or concerns. With its customizable nature and potential to enhance multiple facets of health, intermittent fasting can be a valuable tool in the journey toward improved well-being and longevity.

CHAPTER V

Empowering Women with Intermittent Fasting

5.1: Unveiling Gender-Specific Outcomes – How Women Thrive with Intermittent Fasting

Women experience distinct physiological changes throughout their lives due to hormonal fluctuations. These variations can impact how women respond to intermittent fasting:

Hormonal Differences and Balance: Women experience hormonal fluctuations throughout their menstrual cycle, which can significantly influence how they respond to intermittent fasting. During the follicular phase (pre-ovulation), women generally have higher insulin sensitivity, making fasting more manageable. On the other hand, during the luteal phase (post-ovulation), hormonal changes may increase hunger and make fasting more challenging.

However, the impact of intermittent fasting on hormonal balance should be noticed. Intermittent fasting can help regulate hormonal imbalances in women, promoting more consistent hormone levels. This, in turn, may improve symptoms associated with PMS and perimenopause, providing relief for women during these phases of their cycle.

By understanding these hormonal differences and leveraging the benefits of intermittent fasting on hormonal balance, women can customize their fasting approach to align with their menstrual cycle and overall well-being. This mindful and empowered approach allows women to harness the transformative potential of intermittent fasting while supporting their unique physiological needs at different stages of their cycle.

Caloric Needs: Women typically have lower calorie requirements than men due to differences in body composition and metabolism. Women must ensure they consume adequate nutrients during their eating windows to support their overall health and energy levels.

Fertility Considerations: For women trying to conceive, intermittent fasting should be cautiously approached. Extreme fasting or caloric restriction may impact fertility, and it is essential to prioritize adequate nutrition during this phase.

Menopause and Beyond: Intermittent fasting can be especially beneficial during menopause, as it may help manage weight, reduce hot flashes, and improve insulin sensitivity.

Bone Health: Women are at higher risk of osteoporosis, and prolonged fasting without adequate nutrient intake may increase this risk. Ensuring sufficient calcium, vitamin D, and other bone-supporting nutrients is crucial for women practicing intermittent fasting.

Nurturing the Body: Women often have a nurturing role in society, and it's crucial for women engaging in intermittent fasting to prioritize self-care and listen to their bodies cues.

5.2: Nourishing Well-being – Essential Supplements and Vitamins for Women Over 50

As women age, their nutritional needs evolve, and it becomes crucial to prioritize their health by ensuring adequate intake of essential vitamins and supplements. During intermittent fasting, nourishing the body with vital nutrients is necessary to support overall well-being. This subchapter focuses on recommended supplements and vitamins that benefit women over 50, especially during intermittent fasting, providing insights into their benefits and support.

Multivitamins:
A high-quality multivitamin formulated for women over 50 can be a foundation for overall health. These supplements typically contain essential vitamins and minerals, including vitamin D, calcium, magnesium, and B. Multivitamins can help fill nutritional gaps, support bone health, and boost the immune system.

Vitamin D:
Vitamin D is vital for women over 50, supporting bone health, immune function, and overall well-being. During intermittent fasting, when exposure to sunlight may be limited, a vitamin D supplement can help maintain adequate levels of this essential nutrient.

Calcium:
Calcium is vital for preserving bone mass and avoiding osteoporosis, a condition more common in women as they age. While calcium-rich foods should be part of the diet, a calcium **supplement may be necessary to meet daily requirements, especially for those with limited dairy intake.**

Omega-3 Fatty Acids:
Omega-3 fatty acids, particularly EPA and DHA, play a significant role in heart health and brain function. These essential fats can be found in fatty fish like salmon and mackerel, but a high-quality fish oil supplement can provide the necessary Omega-3s for those with limited fish consumption.

Magnesium:
Magnesium is crucial for muscle function, heart health, and proper nerve function. It can also help alleviate muscle cramps and improve sleep quality, making it beneficial for women over 50, especially during intermittent fasting.

Probiotics:
Probiotics support gut health by promoting the growth of beneficial bacteria. As women age, gut health becomes increasingly essential for digestion and nutrient absorption. A probiotic supplement can help maintain a healthy gut microbiome.

Vitamin B12:
Vitamin B12 is essential for developing red blood cells, neuronal activity, and energy generation. Since B12 is mainly found in animal products, women following a vegetarian or vegan diet may benefit from a B12 supplement.

Coenzyme Q10 (CoQ10):
Coenzyme Q10 is an antioxidant that supports heart health and cellular energy production. As women age, the body's natural production of CoQ10 may decline, making supplementation beneficial.

Collagen:
Collagen is a protein that supports skin elasticity, joint health, and hair strength. As women age, collagen production decreases, and a collagen supplement can help maintain skin health and reduce joint discomfort.

I think speaking with a healthcare provider before beginning new supplements is very important because individual requirements may change depending on health issues and dietary preferences. Additionally, obtaining essential nutrients through a balanced and varied diet should always be the primary focus. Supplements should complement a healthy lifestyle and support the unique needs of women over 50 during their intermittent fasting journey.

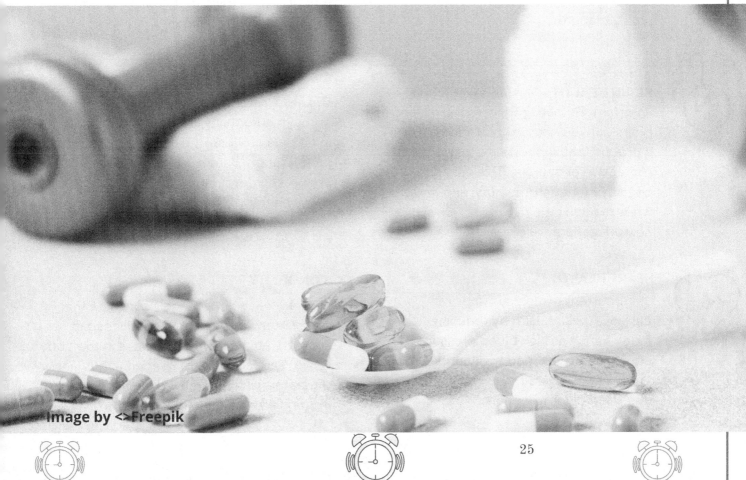

Image by <>Freepik

CHAPTER VI

The Transformative Benefits of Intermittent Fasting

Intermittent fasting is not merely a weight-loss diet; it offers many transformative benefits beyond shedding pounds. In this chapter, we explore the multifaceted impact of fasting on various aspects of health, from inflammation control to cellular detoxification and rejuvenation.

6.1: Beyond Weight Loss – Unraveling the Multifaceted Impact of Fasting

INSULIN SENSITIVITY

Intermittent fasting can improve insulin sensitivity, allowing cells to utilize glucose for energy more effectively.
This helps regulate blood sugar levels, reducing the risk of insulin resistance and type 2 diabetes.

HORMONAL BALANCE

Fasting can positively influence hormone levels, including growth hormone, cortisol, and adiponectin. This hormonal optimization supports various bodily functions, including metabolism, energy regulation, and fat burning.

BRAIN HEALTH

Intermittent fasting triggers the release of brain-derived neurotrophic factor (BDNF), a protein that supports the growth and protection of neurons. This enhances cognitive function, memory, and mood while reducing the risk of neurodegenerative diseases.

CELLULAR REPAIR

Through autophagy, intermittent fasting initiates a process of cellular repair and regeneration. Damaged cells and organelles are broken down, promoting the growth of new, healthy cells and enhancing overall cellular function in neurodegenerative diseases.

HEART HEALTH

Intermittent fasting can improve cardiovascular health by reducing risk factors such as high blood pressure, cholesterol levels, and triglycerides. This, in turn, lowers the risk of heart disease and related complications.

LONGEVITY

Research in animal models suggests that intermittent fasting can extend lifespan and activate longevity pathways in the body. While more studies are needed in humans, the potential for increased longevity is an exciting area of investigation.

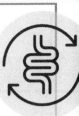

IMMUNE SYSTEM SUPPORT

Fasting has been shown to promote immune system regulation and reduce inflammatory cytokines. This supports a healthy immune response and may reduce the risk of chronic inflammatory conditions.

GUT HEALTH

Intermittent fasting can positively impact the gut microbiome, fostering a balance of beneficial microorganisms that support digestion and overall gut health.

OXIDATIVE STRESS REDUCTION

By promoting autophagy and improving antioxidant defense systems, intermittent fasting can help combat oxidative stress, a key driver of aging and chronic diseases.

6.2: Inflammation Under Control – How Intermittent Fasting Counters Chronic Diseases

Chronic inflammation is at the root of many diseases, including obesity, diabetes, cardiovascular conditions, and neurodegenerative disorders. Intermittent fasting has shown considerable promise in countering chronic inflammation and mitigating the risk of associated diseases:

Reducing Inflammatory Markers: Studies have demonstrated that intermittent fasting can decrease various inflammatory markers, including C-reactive protein (CRP), interleukin-6 (IL-6), and tumor necrosis factor-alpha (TNF-alpha).

Immune System Regulation: Fasting supports a balanced immune response, ensuring the immune system doesn't overreact and cause excessive inflammation.

Autophagy and Inflammation: Autophagy, stimulated by fasting, helps clear out damaged cells and protein aggregates contributing to chronic inflammation.

Antioxidant Defense: Intermittent fasting enhances the body's antioxidant defense mechanisms, reducing oxidative stress and subsequent inflammation.

Impact on Chronic Diseases: By controlling inflammation, intermittent fasting may protect against chronic diseases, including type 2 diabetes, cardiovascular conditions, and neurodegenerative disorders.

6.3: The Inner Cleanse - Cellular Detoxification and Rejuvenation

Cellular detoxification is critical for maintaining cellular health and preventing the accumulation of toxins that can lead to disease. Intermittent fasting promotes the inner cleanse through autophagy, resulting in cellular detoxification and rejuvenation:

Autophagy and Toxin Removal: Autophagy is a natural process that involves the recycling and removing damaged cellular components, including accumulated toxins. This detoxification process helps maintain cellular health and function.

Improved Cellular Function: By clearing out dysfunctional components and allowing new cell growth, intermittent fasting enhances cellular function and supports optimal organ and tissue performance.

Neurological Benefits: Cellular detoxification through autophagy is particularly important for brain health. It helps clear out protein aggregates and dysfunctional mitochondria, reducing the risk of neurodegenerative diseases.

Anti-Aging Effects: Cellular detoxification and rejuvenation contribute to anti-aging effects, as healthier cells lead to improved overall bodily function and reduced risk of age-related diseases.

Weight Loss and Detoxification: As the body breaks down fat during fasting, stored toxins in fat cells are released and eliminated, further promoting detoxification.

Cellular Renewal: Autophagy and cellular detoxification facilitate cellular renewal, promoting the growth of healthy cells and tissues throughout the body.

Incorporating intermittent fasting into your lifestyle can provide transformative benefits, including improved metabolic health, enhanced brain function, reduced inflammation, and cellular detoxification. Understanding these multifaceted impacts empowers you to embrace intermittent fasting as a sustainable and effective dietary approach for long-term well-being and vitality.

CHAPTER VII

Embarking on Your Intermittent Fasting Journey

Intermittent fasting is a transformative dietary approach with immense potential for improving overall health and well-being. As you begin your intermittent fasting journey, this chapter will guide you step-by-step, providing essential information to ensure a smooth and successful start. From understanding different fasting methods to crafting a personalized fasting schedule and optimizing nutrition, you will learn how to embark on your intermittent fasting journey with confidence and mindfulness.

7.1: Ready, Set, Fast! – Step-by-Step Guide to Starting Intermittent Fasting

Before diving into intermittent fasting, it's essential to be prepared mentally and physically for this lifestyle change. In this subchapter, you'll find a comprehensive step-by-step guide to help you ease into intermittent fasting smoothly and effectively.

Educate Yourself: Start by learning about the various intermittent fasting methods, including the 16/8 method, 24-hour fasts, and alternate-day fasting. Understand how each method works, its potential benefits, and its differences.

Set Realistic Goals: Determine your primary objectives for intermittent fasting. Whether it's weight loss, improved energy, better mental clarity, or enhanced overall health, clear and achievable goals will motivate you throughout your journey.

Consult with a Healthcare Professional: If you have any underlying health conditions, take medications, or are pregnant or breastfeeding, consult a healthcare professional before starting intermittent fasting. Your healthcare provider can offer personalized guidance and ensure that intermittent fasting is safe.

Choose the Right Fasting Method: Select the fasting method that aligns best with your lifestyle and preferences. Consider your daily routine, work schedule, and social commitments when making this choice.

Start Gradually: If you're new to fasting, consider easing into it gradually. Begin with shorter fasting periods and extend the fasting window progressively as your body adapts. This approach can help minimize potential discomfort during the transition.

Stay Hydrated: Drink plenty of water throughout fasting to stay hydrated and support your body's detoxification processes.

Listen to Your Body: How your body responds to intermittent fasting. If you experience any adverse effects or feel unwell, consider adjusting your fasting schedule or seeking guidance from a healthcare professional.

Be Patient and Persistent: Like any lifestyle change, intermittent fasting may take time to yield noticeable results. Stay patient and persistent, and trust the process.

7.2: Designing Your Unique Plan – Crafting a Fasting and Feeding Schedule

Designing a fasting and feeding schedule that suits your lifestyle and individual needs is key to a successful intermittent fasting journey. This subchapter teaches you how to create a personalized plan that aligns with your goals and daily activities.

Determine Your Fasting Window: Choose the duration of your fasting window based on your chosen fasting method and daily routine. The fasting window is the time between your last meal and your first meal the following day.

Select Your Feeding Window: Decide on the duration of your feeding window, which is the time when you consume all your daily calories. Ensure that your feeding window allows you to enjoy fulfilling and nutritious meals.

Customize Your Schedule: Tailor your fasting and feeding schedule to fit your daily commitments. You can adjust the timing of your fasting and feeding windows to accommodate work, family, and social activities.

Experiment and Adapt: Finding the ideal fasting schedule may require trial and error. Please be open to experimenting with different fasting and feeding windows until you find out what works best for you.

Plan Your Meals: Prepare balanced and nourishing meals that provide essential nutrients during your feeding window. Focus on whole foods, lean proteins, healthy fats, and fruits and vegetables.

Consider Exercise: If you exercise regularly, consider how your fasting schedule may impact your workouts. Some individuals prefer to exercise during their feeding window to ensure they have enough energy for physical activity.

Be Consistent: Consistency is key to reaping the benefits of intermittent fasting. Stick to your chosen fasting and feeding schedule as consistently as possible.

7.3: Nurturing Well-being – Balancing Nutrition and Intermittent Fasting

Balanced nutrition is fundamental to supporting your health and well-being during intermittent fasting. In this subchapter, you'll discover how to maintain a healthy and nourishing diet that complements your fasting lifestyle.

Prioritize Nutrient-Dense Foods: Choose nutrients that provide essential vitamins, minerals, and antioxidants. Include a variety of colorful fruits and vegetables, whole grains, lean proteins, and healthy fats in your meals.

Avoid Processed Foods: Minimize the intake of processed and sugary foods, as they can negatively impact your health and undermine the benefits of intermittent fasting.

Stay Mindful of Portion Sizes: Pay attention to portion sizes during your feeding window to ensure you consume the right calories and nutrients for your body's needs.

Stay Hydrated: Drink enough water throughout the day to support your body's functions and reduce the risk of dehydration during fasting.

Consider Supplements: If needed, consider adding supplements to fill potential nutrient gaps in your diet. Consult with a healthcare professional to determine which supplements are appropriate for you.

Monitor Your Progress: Keep track of your fasting journey and monitor how you feel, any changes in your body, and your overall well-being. This self-awareness will help you adjust and continue on a path of growth and improvement.

Seek Support: Connect with others on an intermittent fasting journey or seek guidance from online communities and resources. Sharing experiences and tips can be motivating and helpful as you navigate your fasting lifestyle.

By following these guidelines and nurturing your well-being through balanced nutrition, you can make the most of your intermittent fasting journey and experience its transformative benefits for long-term health and vitality.

CHAPTER VIII

Illuminating the Future of Intermittent Fasting

Intermittent fasting has garnered significant attention in the scientific community and among health enthusiasts. As researchers continue to explore its potential, discoveries and insights, emerge, shedding light on the future of this transformative dietary approach. This chapter delves into the latest research and developments surrounding intermittent fasting, explores its integration into a long-term lifestyle, and examines the powerful synergy between exercise and fasting for maximizing results.

8.1: A Scientific Frontier – Promising Research and Groundbreaking Discoveries

Intermittent fasting has become a subject of intense scientific inquiry, with researchers striving to uncover the underlying mechanisms and comprehensive health effects. This subchapter delves into some of the most promising research and groundbreaking discoveries surrounding intermittent fasting.

Cellular Autophagy: One of the key areas of interest in intermittent fasting research is cellular autophagy, a natural process that helps cells remove damaged components and regenerate. Intermittent fasting has been found to enhance autophagy, promoting cellular health and potentially reducing the risk of age-related diseases.

Hormonal Regulation: Research has demonstrated that intermittent fasting can influence various hormones, such as insulin, ghrelin, and leptin, which play crucial roles in metabolism, hunger regulation, and fat storage.

Understanding these hormonal responses is vital for optimizing the benefits of fasting.

Brain Health and Cognitive Function: Recent studies have indicated that intermittent fasting may have neuroprotective effects, supporting brain health and cognitive function. It has been linked to increased brain-derived neurotrophic factor (BDNF) production, a protein that promotes brain cell growth and mental performance.

Longevity Pathways: Some animal studies have suggested that intermittent fasting can activate specific longevity pathways, such as the sirtuin genes. These pathways have been associated with extended lifespan and protection against age-related diseases.

Gut Microbiome: Intermittent fasting may also influence the composition of the gut microbiome, the community of microorganisms in the digestive tract. A balanced and diverse gut microbiome is linked to improved digestion, immune function, and overall health.

Disease Prevention: Research on intermittent fasting's potential to prevent and manage chronic diseases such as diabetes, heart disease, and certain cancers is ongoing. Early findings show promise, but more extensive, long-term human studies are needed to draw definitive conclusions.

Psychological Well-being: Beyond physical health, intermittent fasting may positively impact mental and emotional well-being. Some studies suggest intermittent fasting improves mood, reduces stress, and enhances mental clarity.

8.2: Strengthening Health for Life – Embracing Intermittent Fasting as a Way of Life

Intermittent fasting is not just a short-term diet plan; it is a lifestyle that can empower you to take charge of your health and well-being for the long haul. As you become more familiar with the many benefits and transformative effects of intermittent fasting, you may naturally embrace it as a way of life. This subchapter delves into why intermittent fasting can be a robust and sustainable approach to health, providing you with the tools and knowledge to make it an integral part of your lifestyle.

A Lifestyle Rooted in Tradition:

Intermittent fasting is not a new concept. It has ancient roots in various cultures and has been practiced for centuries to optimize health and spirituality. In modern times, the resurgence of intermittent fasting is driven by a growing body of scientific research that supports its positive effects on health, longevity, and disease prevention.

Embracing Flexibility and Freedom:

One of the key reasons intermittent fasting can be adopted as a lifelong lifestyle is its flexibility. Unlike strict and rigid diets, intermittent fasting offers different methods to be customized to fit your preferences, schedule, and health goals. Whether you prefer the simplicity of the 16/8 method or the occasional 24-hour fast, intermittent fasting allows you to choose what works best.

Sustainable Weight Management:

Many people initially turn to intermittent fasting for its weight loss benefits, but its impact on weight management goes beyond shedding a few pounds. Intermittent fasting helps regulate appetite hormones, leading to healthier eating patterns and reduced calorie intake. By promoting fat loss while preserving muscle mass, intermittent fasting supports sustainable weight management, making it easier to maintain a healthy weight in the long run.

Empowering Hormonal Balance:

For women, intermittent fasting can be incredibly empowering in promoting hormonal balance. It helps regulate hormone levels, reducing the symptoms associated with PMS and perimenopause. Understanding the hormonal differences throughout the menstrual cycle can guide women in tailoring their fasting approach for optimal results at different stages.

Enhanced Brain Health and Cognitive Function:

Intermittent fasting's impact on brain health and cognitive function is another compelling reason to embrace it as a lifestyle. By promoting neuroplasticity and stimulating the production of brain-derived neurotrophic factor (BDNF), intermittent fasting supports improved memory, focus, and overall cognitive performance.

Long-Term Disease Prevention:

Adopting intermittent fasting as a way of life can significantly contribute to long-term disease prevention. Its effects on reducing inflammation, improving insulin sensitivity, and supporting a healthy heart and cardiovascular system can lower the risk of chronic diseases such as type 2 diabetes, heart disease, and neurodegenerative conditions.

Emotional and Psychological Well-being:

Intermittent fasting positively impacts physical health and emotional and psychological well-being. Many individuals report feeling empowered, increased self-discipline, and improved mood and mental clarity while practicing intermittent fasting.

Building a Sustainable Routine:

Building a sustainable routine that works for you is essential to embrace intermittent fasting as a lifelong lifestyle. Gradually incorporating intermittent fasting into your daily life, understanding your body's signals, and listening to its needs will help you create a harmonious balance between fasting and feeding.

Embracing intermittent fasting as a way of life requires patience, self-compassion, and a commitment to long-term well-being. As you embark on this journey, remember that everyone's experience is unique, and what matters most is finding a sustainable approach that supports your health, happiness, and personal growth. By making intermittent fasting a part of your lifestyle, you can unlock its transformative potential and experience its numerous benefits for a healthier and more fulfilling life.

8.3: Synergy of Strength – Maximizing Results with Exercise and Fasting

Intermittent fasting has garnered significant attention in the scientific community and among health enthusiasts. As researchers continue to explore its potential, discoveries and insights, emerge, shedding light on the future of this transformative dietary approach. This chapter delves into the latest research and developments surrounding intermittent fasting, explores its integration into a long-term lifestyle, and examines the powerful synergy between exercise and fasting for maximizing results.

Fasting and Exercise Timing: Consider the timing of your workouts about your fasting and feeding windows. Some individuals prefer exercising during their feeding window to ensure they have enough energy for physical activity.

Benefits of Fasted Exercise: Exercising during fasting may promote greater fat burning, as the body relies on stored fat for energy. It can also boost cellular autophagy, enhancing cellular repair and regeneration.

Listen to Your Body: Pay attention to how your body responds to exercise during fasting. While some individuals may thrive with fasted workouts, others may feel better with a small meal or snack before exercising.

Stay Hydrated: Drink sufficient water before, during, and after exercise, especially when fasting, to maintain hydration and support performance.

Fueling Post-Workout: After exercising, consume a balanced meal rich in protein, healthy fats, and carbohydrates to support muscle recovery and replenish glycogen stores.

Types of Exercise: Intermittent fasting can complement various forms of exercise, including cardiovascular workouts, strength training, yoga, and high-intensity interval training (HIIT). You can choose activities that align with your fitness goals and preferences.

Rest and Recovery: Allow your body adequate time to rest and recover between workouts, as recovery is crucial for muscle repair and overall well-being.

By understanding the latest research, embracing intermittent fasting as a lifestyle, and synergizing it with exercise, you can unlock the full potential of this transformative approach to health and well-being. Through mindfulness, consistency, and adaptability, you can illuminate your path toward a healthier and more vibrant future with intermittent fasting.

CHAPTER IX

Mastering Hunger and Satiety Strategies to Overcome Cravings and Achieve Satisfying Meals

9.1: Understanding Hunger Attacks – Overcoming Cravings with Intermittent Fasting

Hunger attacks can strike any time, driven by various factors such as anxiety, boredom, hormonal changes, or external triggers. These attacks often lead to consuming processed, high-calorie, or sugary foods, disrupting the progress of intermittent fasting. To counteract these challenges and ensure successful fasting periods, it is essential to understand the underlying causes of hunger and implement effective strategies.

Managing Blood Sugar Levels:
Frequent fluctuations in blood sugar levels can trigger intense hunger. To stabilize blood glucose, eat balanced meals that include whole grains, protein, healthy fats, and fiber. Avoid high-glycemic foods that cause rapid spikes and crashes in blood sugar. Eating smaller, more frequent daily meals can help prevent extreme hunger.

Stay Hydrated:
Drinking an ample amount of water throughout the day can help curb hunger. Hydration can create a sense of fullness and reduce the urge to snack unnecessarily. Before meals, drink water or herbal tea to promote satiety.

Mindful Eating:
Practice mindful eating by savoring each bite and chewing food thoroughly. This approach allows the brain to recognize fullness signals accurately, preventing overeating. Eating slowly also enhances the enjoyment of food and aids in better digestion.

Opt for Warm Dishes:
Studies suggest hot foods promote a more incredible feeling of fullness than cold foods. Consider heating dishes initially planned to be eaten out to enhance satisfaction and reduce overall consumption.

Distract from Temptations:
Avoid keeping unhealthy snacks readily available. Store tempting treats out of sight and replace them with healthier options like fruits, nuts, or vegetables. This simple change can positively impact eating habits and reduce mindless snacking.

Address Stress and Anxiety:
Stress and anxiety can trigger emotional eating, leading to overconsumption of calorie-dense foods. Engage in stress-reducing activities like meditation, yoga, or spending time in nature to manage stress effectively. Additionally, consider incorporating foods rich in vitamin B6, folic acid, and tryptophan into the diet to support serotonin production and promote well-being.

Prioritize Satiating Foods:
Begin main meals with a hearty salad to help reduce overall hunger. Choose dishes that require more chewing, like raw vegetables, to increase meal duration and provide a greater sense of fullness.

Quality Sleep:
Adequate sleep is essential for hunger regulation and overall health. Lack of sleep can disrupt hunger hormones, leading to increased appetite and cravings. Strive for 7-9 hours of sleep per night to support the body's natural regulatory processes.

9.2: Habits for Healthy Weight Management – Tips to Lose Weight without Starving

Intermittent fasting can be a powerful tool for weight management, but it is essential to complement it with healthy habits to achieve sustainable results. Please emphasize the following strategies alongside intermittent fasting for effective and satisfying weight loss.

Portion Control:
Moderation is key. Focus on reducing portion sizes rather than eliminating entire food groups. Smaller portions can help maintain satisfaction while controlling calorie intake.

01

Opt for Real Foods:
Choose nutrient-dense, whole foods over refined and processed options. Avoid foods with added sugars, unhealthy fats, and artificial additives.

02

Limit Sugar Intake:
Reduce sugar consumption as it contributes to weight gain and various health issues. Choose products with little to no added sugars, and opt for natural sweeteners in moderation.

03

Hydration:
Stay adequately hydrated by drinking at least two liters of water daily. Water helps cleanse the body, supports metabolism, and reduces feelings of hunger when consumed before meals.

04

Mindful Eating:
Practice mindful eating to become more aware of hunger cues and satiety signals. Avoid distractions while eating and focus on enjoying the flavors and textures of each meal.

05

By incorporating these practices into your intermittent fasting journey, you can overcome hunger attacks, improve satiety, and achieve your weight management goals while embracing intermittent fasting as a sustainable way of life.

CHAPTER X

Activating Your Body
The Vital Role of Physical
Activity in Intermittent Fasting

10.1: Synergy of Exercise and Fasting – Unveiling the Benefits of Physical Activity

Physical activity is a crucial component of a healthy lifestyle, and when combined with intermittent fasting, it can enhance the overall benefits and results. Exercise not only aids in weight management but also offers numerous other advantages that synergize with intermittent fasting to promote general well-being.

Enhanced Fat Burning:
When you engage in physical activity during fasting, your body utilizes stored fat as an energy source, accelerating fat-burning. This combination can lead to more significant improvements in body composition.

Improved Insulin Sensitivity:
Exercise, particularly aerobic activities like walking, running, or cycling, can improve insulin sensitivity. This means your body becomes more efficient at using insulin to regulate blood sugar levels, reducing the risk of insulin resistance and type 2 diabetes.

Muscle Preservation:
Integrating resistance training into your exercise routine helps preserve and build muscle mass, even during periods of calorie restriction. Maintaining muscle is essential for a higher metabolic rate and overall strength.

Boosted Metabolism:
Regular exercise stimulates the metabolism, leading to increased calorie expenditure even at rest. This metabolic boost complements the effects of intermittent fasting and supports weight loss and maintenance.

Enhanced Brain Health:
Physical activity positively affects cognitive function and mood, reducing stress and anxiety. This mental well-being aligns with the clarity and focus often experienced during fasting.

Cardiovascular Health:
Exercise supports heart health by improving cardiovascular fitness, reducing blood pressure, and enhancing circulation. Combined with the potential cardiovascular benefits of intermittent fasting, this duo promotes a healthy heart.

10.2: Finding Your Fitness Flow – Recommended Physical Activities for Home Workouts

Exercising at home provides a convenient and effective way to stay active, especially when complementing intermittent fasting. Here is a list of exercises that require minimal equipment and can be easily performed at home:

- **Bodyweight Exercises:**

Push-ups: Target the chest, shoulders, and triceps.

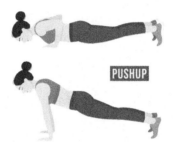

Squats: Engage the lower body, including the glutes, quads, and hamstrings.

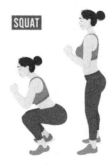

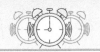
Lunges: Work the legs and improve balance.

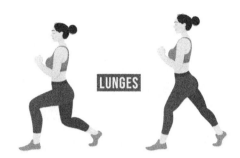

Planks Row: Strengthen the core, shoulders, and back.

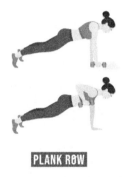

- **Cardio Workouts:**

Jumping Jacks: Elevate heart rate and improve cardiovascular endurance.

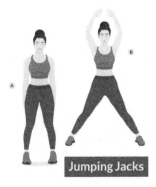

High Stepping/Knees: Perform in place by alternating lifting knees towards the chest.

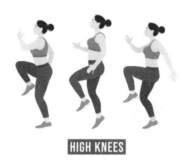

Jump-Squat: A fun and effective cardio workout with minimal space required.

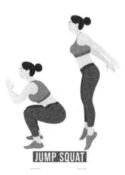

- **Yoga and Stretching:**

Cat Cow: Prevent back pain and maintain a healthy spine, help improve posture and balance.

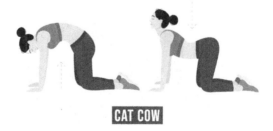

Child's Pose: Relieve tension in the lower back and hips.

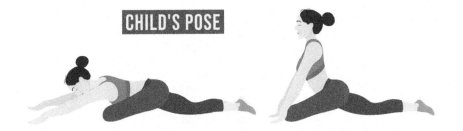

Cobra Pose: Strengthen the back and open up the chest.

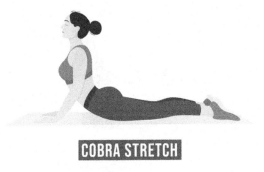

- **Resistance Bands:**

Cactus Arms: Target the biceps using resistance bands, if you have any, for added challenge.

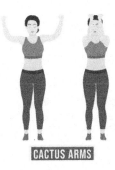

Dumbbell Tricep Extensions: Work your triceps by extending your arms overhead with weights

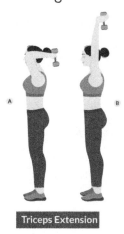

Glute Bridge: Engage the glutes and hamstrings with the band looped around the thighs.

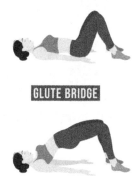

- **HIIT Workouts:**

  Burpees: Full-body exercise that combines a squat, plank, and jump.

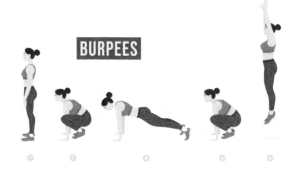

Cross Mountain Climbers: Dynamic exercise targeting the core and shoulders.

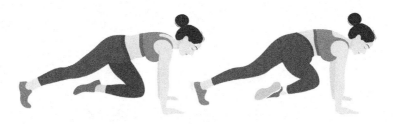

High-intensity interval training (HIIT): Alternate bursts of intense activity and short periods of rest to increase heart rate and burn calories. Below are work out patterns you might do

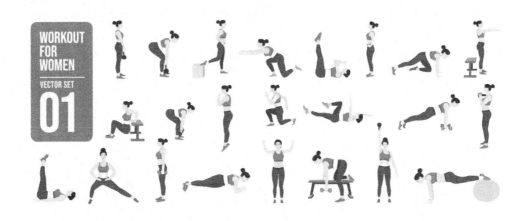

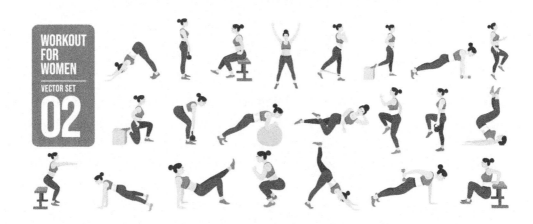

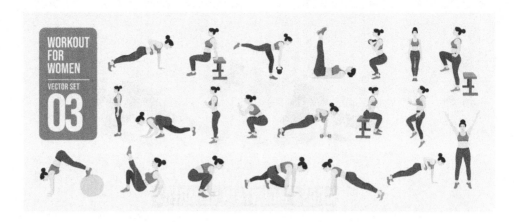

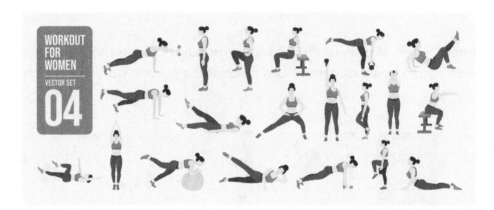

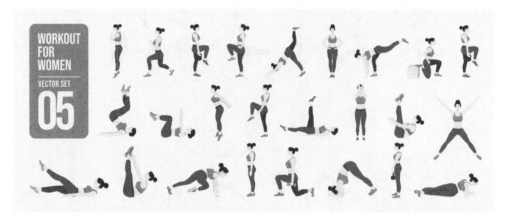

Remember to warm up before exercising and cool down afterward. Start with exercises that match your fitness level and gradually progress to more challenging routines. Always listen to your body and consult with a healthcare professional before beginning a new exercise regimen, especially if you have any medical conditions or concerns.

By incorporating physical activity into your intermittent fasting lifestyle, you can optimize your health, amplify the benefits of fasting, and enjoy an active and energized life.

CHAPTER XI

Nourishing Your Body Food Choices for Intermittent Fasting Success

11.1: Foods to Embrace – Nourishing Your Body During Intermittent Fasting

During intermittent fasting, the foods you consume during your feeding windows support your overall well-being. Focus on incorporating nutrient-dense foods that provide essential nutrients and satisfy you.

Avocado: Rich in healthy fats, avocados are an excellent meal addition. They promote feelings of fullness and satisfaction, helping you stay on track with your fasting schedule.

Fish: Incorporate fish into your diet at least twice a week. Fish is a valuable source of protein and healthy fats, such as omega-3 fatty acids, contributing to heart health and brain function.

Sweet Potato: Opt for baked or roasted sweet potatoes, which provide a good source of healthy fibers and carbohydrates. These nutrients contribute to a sense of satiety, making them an ideal choice for intermittent fasting.

Eggs: Eggs are a protein powerhouse and contain essential nutrients supporting muscle mass and energy levels during fasting.

Nuts and Seeds: Nuts and seeds, such as almonds, cashews, and chia seeds, are rich in calories, proteins, and fibers. They make excellent snacks that can help you stay full between meals.

Whole Grains: Choose whole grains like brown rice, quinoa, and oats over refined grains. Whole grains are rich in healthy carbohydrates and fiber, optimizing metabolism and aiding in weight management.

Probiotic Foods: Yogurt, kefir, and fermented milk products support a healthy gut. They contain probiotics that promote proper digestion and overall gut health.

Cruciferous Vegetables: Broccoli, cauliflower, and Brussels sprouts are fiber-rich vegetables that promote feelings of fullness and contribute to intestinal health.

Foods Rich in Flavonoids: Include foods like berries, apples, and citrus fruits. Flavonoids have been linked to decreased BMI over time and provide various health benefits.

11.2: Foods to Avoid – Making Smart Choices for Intermittent Fasting

Avoiding certain foods during your feeding windows is essential for making the most of your intermittent fasting journey. Steer clear of processed and unhealthy options that may disrupt your fasting progress.

Sugary Treats: Say no to candies, sweets, and desserts loaded with sugar. High sugar intake is linked to weight gain and various health issues.

Processed Cookies: Skip packaged and processed cookies, which are high in unhealthy fats, sugar, and empty calories.

Frozen or Canned Foods: Processed frozen or canned foods often contain added preservatives and high sodium levels, negatively impacting your health and well-being.

Ready Sauces: Many ready-made sauces and condiments contain hidden sugars and unhealthy fats. Opt for homemade alternatives or use herbs and spices to flavor your dishes.

Whole Dairy Products: Full-fat dairy products can be high in calories and saturated fats. Choose low-fat or plant-based alternatives if needed.

Refined Cereals: Avoid refined cereals like white rice and white bread. Opt for whole grain options that provide more nutrients and promote stable blood sugar levels.

Fried Snacks: Avoid fried snacks, which are high in unhealthy fats and can lead to weight gain.

Excessive Salt and Sugar: Minimize your use of salt and sugar when preparing meals. Too much sodium can lead to water retention and excessive sugar consumption is linked to various health issues.

Embrace nutrient-dense foods, avoid processed choices, and balanced meals to support your health during intermittent fasting. Listen to your body, stay hydrated, and seek professional advice for personalized guidance.

RECIPES
BREAKFASTS

1. PERFECT HARD-BOILED EGGS IN THE EASIEST MANNER

 15 minutes 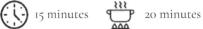 20 minutes 2 servings

NUTRIENT VALUE:
PER SERVING

 71 kcal

 0 g

 6 g

 4 g

Ingredients

- 6 large eggs
- Water (enough to cover the eggs)

Directions

- The eggs should be arranged in a single layer in a medium saucepan.
- Pour in just enough water to cover the eggs in the pan by about 1 inch.
- Put the pot on the burner and turn the heat to high.
- Water is brought to a boil.
- When the water boils, quickly turn off the heat and cover the pan.
- Give the eggs 18 to 20 minutes to rest in the boiling water.
- Prepare a dish of ice water while the eggs are waiting.
- After the specified amount of time has passed, gently pour the hot water out of the saucepan while holding it at an angle that will enable it to escape.
- Place the eggs in the bowl of cold water, where they should sit for a minute or two before being peeled.

2. MIX TRAIL

 2 minutes 0 minutes 6 servings

NUTRIENT VALUE:
WHOLE RECIPE

 371 kcal

 35 g

 10 g

 24 g

Ingredients

- 1 cup almonds (230 g)
- 1 cup sunflower seeds (230 g)
- 1 cup raisins (230 g)
- 3/4 cup dried apricot
- 2 ounces of flaked coconut (optional, 60 g)
- 1/4 cup chocolate or carob chips (60 g)

Directions

- 1. Combine each item in a large container.
- To thoroughly combine the trail mix, cover the container and shake it.
- Store the trail mix in an airtight container.
- Refrigerate or freeze the trail mix to preserve its freshness and vital fatty acid characteristics.

3. BOWL OF SAVORY OATS

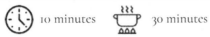 10 minutes   30 minutes   4 servings

Ingredients

NUTRIENT VALUE:
WHOLE RECIPE

460 kcal

56 g

19 g

17 g

- 1/2 lb halved Brussels sprouts (225 g)
- Butternut squash, chopped, 1 lb (450 g)
- 1 tbsp/15 ml virgin olive oil
- Salt (to taste, divided)
- Black pepper (to taste, divided)
- 1 tbsp unsalted butter (15 g)
- 1/2 cup finely chopped onion (120 g)
- 2 cups Quaker Old-Fashioned Oats (450 g)
- 2 cups water (450 ml)
- 2 ounces of shredded Sharp Cheddar cheese (120 g)
- 4 quail eggs
- 2 cooked turkey bacon strips, crumbled

Directions

- Set the oven's temperature to 400°F (204°C).
- Using parchment paper, line a large baking sheet.
- Toss the butternut squash, Brussels sprouts, finely sliced onion, black pepper, 1/2 teaspoon of salt, and olive oil in a large mixing basin until everything is well covered.
- Transfer the prepared baking sheet with the veggies, and bake for 20 to 22 minutes until the vegetables are soft and golden brown.
- Melt the butter in a medium saucepan over medium heat, then toast the oats for 30 seconds while the veggies roast.
- Bring the pot's contents to a boil after adding water. Oats should be cooked for 8 to 10 minutes on low heat or until they become thick, adding extra water as necessary.
- Finishes the remaining salt and pepper to the oats before incorporating the cheese shreds.
- Cook the quail eggs sunny-side up or over easy in a large oiled nonstick pan.
- Pour the oats into bowls, add the roasted vegetables, a quail egg, and the turkey bacon crumbles, and serve.

4. THE BUDDHA BOWL

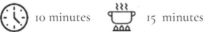 10 minutes   15 minutes   2 servings

Ingredients

- 2 poached pastured eggs
- 2 precooked Paleo sausages (spicy lamb sausage)
- 2 1/2 cups riced cauliflower (250 g)
- 2 tbsp grass-fed ghee for cooking (30 ml)
- 1 avocado, sliced
- Sliced cucumber

- two handfuls of organic leafy greens
- a lemon wedge, fresh herbs, sliced chiles, sliced spring onions, salt, and pepper (to taste) for garnish.

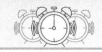
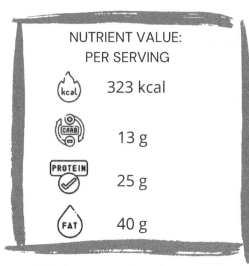

**NUTRIENT VALUE:
PER SERVING**

kcal   323 kcal

CARB   13 g

PROTEIN   25 g

FAT   40 g

Directions

- 2 tbsp of grass-fed ghee should be melted in a frying pan over medium heat.
- Cook the riced cauliflower in the pan until it reaches your preferred doneness.
- Place the leafy greens in a big dish or on a platter once they have been softly steamed.
- Over the lush greens, plate the cauliflower rice.
- Sausages should be reheated in the same frying pan.
- While the sausages are warming up, add the sliced avocado, cucumber, and poached eggs to the cauliflower rice and leafy leaves.

- Add the warmed sausages to the bowl containing the remaining ingredients.
- Add a wedge of lemon, fresh herbs, chile slices, and spring onion slices to the dish as a garnish. Add salt and pepper to taste.
- Serve and enjoy!

5. PANCAKES WITH KETO COCONUT FLOUR

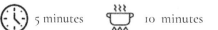 5 minutes   10 minutes   3 servings

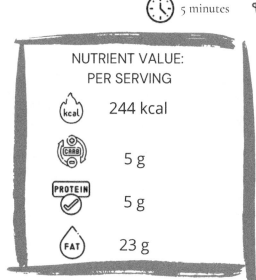

**NUTRIENT VALUE:
PER SERVING**

kcal   244 kcal

CARB   5 g

PROTEIN   5 g

FAT   23 g

Ingredients

- 8 tbsp. (50g) coconut flour
- 1 pinch (3g) baking soda
- 1 tbsp (10ml) melted coconut oil
- 4 organic, pasture-raised eggs, room temp.
- 1/2 tsp (3ml) vanilla extract
- 1 pinch (3g) cinnamon, Ceylon
- 1 cup (250g) Coconut cream (the thick, unsweetened portion of canned coconut cream)
- 8 tbsp. (120ml) stevia-free almond milk
- 1 pinch (2g) Pink salt
- Ghee or coconut oil made from grass-fed cows

Directions

- All ingredients—except the ghee—should be placed in a powerful blender and blended well, scraping down the sides as necessary.
- In a medium skillet, heat the ghee until it completely covers the bottom of the pan.
- Add half of the batter to the pan once it is heated.
- The batter should be cooked until golden brown on one side before turning it over and until golden brown on the other (thicker pancakes will take longer to cook). Cook until no batter is left, then set aside.
- Serve warm pancakes of coconut flour with fruit, grass-fed ghee, or other keto-friendly toppings.

6. PIZZA KETO FOR BREAKFAST (DAIRY-FREE)

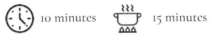 10 minutes   15 minutes   2 servings

Ingredients

- 1 lb (450g) cauliflower, grated
- 1/4 cup coconut flour
- 4 eggs,
- 1 pinch (3g) salt
- 2 tbsp (15g) psyllium husk powder (Use a brand without mold, like this one.)
- Add smoked salmon, avocado, herbs, spinach, and olive oil as toppings (see post for further ideas).

Directions

- The oven should be set to 350°F (176°C).
- A pizza tray or a sheet pan should be lined with parchment paper.

NUTRIENT VALUE: PER SERVING

 454 kcal

 26 g

 22 g

 31 g

- In a mixing bowl, combine all the ingredients—aside from the toppings—and stir thoroughly. Give coconut flour and psyllium husk five minutes to thicken and absorb the liquid.
- Carefully pour the morning pizza foundation onto the pan. Using your hands, shape it into a round, uniform pizza crust.
- Cook for 15 minutes or until well heated through and golden brown.
- The morning pizza should be removed from the oven and topped with your favorite ingredients. Serve warm.

7. COOKIES WITH COLLAGEN FOR BREAKFAST

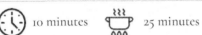 10 minutes   25 minutes   4 servings

Ingredients

- 2 eggs
- 16 tbsp. (120g) almond flour
- 16 tbsp. (120g) shredded coconut
- 16 tbsp. (120g) almonds, sliced
- 16 tbsp. (120g) toasted pecans
- 16 tbsp. (120g) pumpkin seeds
- 8 tbsp. (120g) chocolate chips (sugar-free)
- 1/3 cup (75g) toasted almond butter
- 1/3 cup (75g) granulated monk fruit-erythritol blend
- 2 tbsp (30g) ground flax meal
- 2 tbsp (7g) Bulletproof Collagen Protein in Vanilla
- 2 tsp (20g) cinnamon
- 2 tsp (20g) ginger powder
- 1 tsp (15ml) vanilla extract

NUTRIENT VALUE: PER SERVING

 289 kcal

 17 g

 8 g

 29 g

Directions

- Set the oven's temperature to 350°F (176°C).
- Using parchment paper, line two baking pans.
- All cookie ingredients should be combined in a mixing bowl.
- Make balls out of the mixture by rolling them in coconut oil. Press them into flat, even cookies before placing them on baking trays prepared with parchment paper.
- Bake the baking tray for 20 to 25 minutes or until golden and well done.
- The cookies should be taken out of the oven and let to cool.
- Serve your breakfast with steaming Bulletproof Coffee for a keto-friendly meal!

8. SMOKED SALMON BREAKFAST SANDWICH

 5 minutes 10 minutes 4 servings

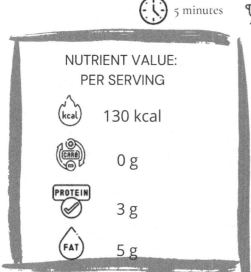

NUTRIENT VALUE:
PER SERVING

(kcal) 130 kcal

(CARB) 0 g

(PROTEIN) 3 g

(FAT) 5 g

Ingredients

- 1/4 cup (60ml) coconut oil
- 8 slices of your choice of sandwich vessel (like Cauliflower Sandwich Thins)
- 4 oz (110g) smoked salmon
- 8 oz (225g) fresh spinach
- 2 whole pasture-raised eggs or 1/4 cup (60g) organic powdered eggs
- 1/4 cup (60ml) water
- 2 garlic cloves or 1 tbsp (7g) garlic powder
- Juice of half a lemon

Directions

- If you're using powdered eggs, hydrate them in water first.
- Allow for a 5-minute resting period after stirring.
- Meanwhile, heat the burner to medium.
- Heat 2 tbsp (30ml) coconut oil in a pan.
- Toast both sides of the sandwich bread.
- Mince the garlic cloves while the bread is browning.
- Add the remaining 2 tbsp (30 ml) of coconut oil to the pan once the slices have been roasted.
- For one to two minutes, cook the garlic.
- Spinach is now added. Cook the spinach for 2 to 3 minutes or until it wilts.
- Eggs are added. Cook for 2 to 3 minutes while gently stirring until set.
- Add a squeeze of lemon juice to the end.
- Put the toasted bread on the smoked salmon and garlic spinach scramble.
- Serve and enjoy!

9. SCRAMBLED EGGS BREAKFAST

 2 minutes 5 minutes 1 servings

NUTRIENT VALUE:
PER SERVING

 263 kcal

 1 g

 5 g

 5 g

Ingredients

- 1 big egg
- 4 tbsp. (60g) egg whites
- 1/2 cup (60g) cheddar cheese, shredded
- 1/2 small avocado (about 15g), sliced
- 1/2 cup (120g) thinly sliced mushrooms

Directions

- Egg and egg whites should be well mixed in a bowl.
- Spray cooking spray onto a pan and heat it to medium heat.
- When the egg mixture is no longer runny, fry it into the skillet.
- In a separate skillet, sauté the mushrooms with butter-flavored cooking spray until soft.
- Sprinkle the shredded cheddar cheese on the cooked eggs and let it melt.
- Top the scrambled eggs with sautéed mushrooms, avocado slices, and additional shredded cheese if desired.

10. LOW-CARB ENGLISH BREAKFAST

 5 minutes 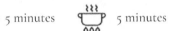 5 minutes 1 servings

NUTRIENT VALUE:
PER SERVING

 690 kcal

 0 g

 2 g

 5 g

Ingredients

- 1 large egg
- 0.7 oz (20g) bacon
- 2 sausages
- 1.06 oz (30g) mushrooms
- 0.5 small avocado (about 1.06 oz or 30g), sliced
- 1 roasted tomato
- 1 cup (30g) wilted spinach

Directions

- Cook the bacon, sausages, mushrooms, and tomato according to your preference.
- Remove high-carbohydrate products like bread and hash browns from the usual English breakfast.
- Arrange the cooked items on a plate and top with sliced avocado and wilted spinach.

11. THE FRENCH OMELET

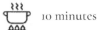 10 minutes   10 minutes   10 minutes   3 servings

Ingredients

- 3 big eggs
- 4 big egg whites
- 1/4 cup (75 ml) fat-free milk
- 1 pinch (2g) pepper
- 1 pinch (2g) salt
- 75g well-cooked cubed ham
- 1/4 cup (15g) finely sliced onion
- 1/2 tsp (3g) chopped green pepper
- 2.65 ounce (75g) reduced-fat cheddar cheese, shredded

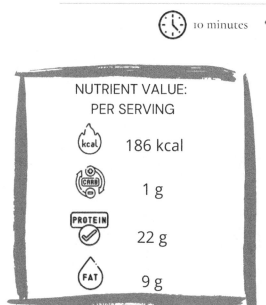

NUTRIENT VALUE:
PER SERVING

kcal 186 kcal

CARB 1 g

PROTEIN 22 g

FAT 9 g

Directions

- Combine the milk, pepper, salt, egg yolks, and egg whites in a mixing bowl.
- Spray cooking spray into a 10-inch skillet and heat it over medium-low heat.
- The skillet will now contain the egg mixture.
- Push the cooked sections towards the center as the eggs set at the edges, allowing uncooked eggs to flow underneath.
- When the eggs have thickened, top half with ham, onion, green pepper, and shredded cheese.
- Fold the omelet in half and cut it into serving portions.

12. FRITTATA WITH FETA

 10 minutes   15 minutes   15 minutes   3 servings

Ingredients

- 1 green onion, finely sliced
- 1 garlic clove, minced
- 2 big eggs
- 2.65 ounces (120g) egg replacer
- 1/4 cup (60g) crumbled feta cheese (divided)
- 1 cup (100g) chopped plum tomato
- 4 thin avocado slices, peeled
- 2 tbsp (30g) reduced-fat sour cream

NUTRIENT VALUE:
PER SERVING

kcal 203 kcal

CARB 5 g

PROTEIN 17 g

FAT 12 g

Directions

- A 6-inch nonstick pan that has been lightly greased is heated over medium heat.
- Green onion slices and garlic cloves in minced form should be cooked till tender.
- Combine the eggs, egg substitute, and half of the feta cheese in a mixing dish.

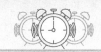

- The egg mixture should instantly solidify at the edges after being poured into the pan.
- The frittata should be cooked and covered for 4–6 minutes or until almost set.
- Top with the remaining feta cheese and tomato slices.
- For 2-3 minutes, or until the eggs are fully formed, cook the frittata with the lid on.
- Before serving, let the frittata five minutes to rest.
- Serve with avocado slices and a dollop of reduced-fat sour cream.

13. FRITTATA WITH BACON AND ASPARAGUS

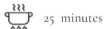 10 minutes 25 minutes 6 servings

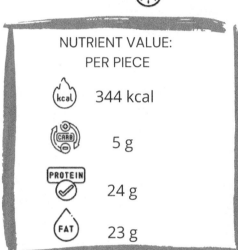

NUTRIENT VALUE:
PER PIECE

344 kcal

5 g

24 g

23 g

Ingredients

- 12.35 oz (350g) bacon
- 15.87 oz (450g) fresh asparagus, sliced (cut into 1/2-inch pieces)
- 8.82 oz (250g) finely chopped onion
- 2 minced garlic cloves
- 10 large eggs, beaten
- 2.12 oz (60g) parsley, minced
- 0.07 oz (2g) seasoned salt
- 0.04 oz (1g) pepper
- 1 large, thinly sliced tomato
- 8.82 oz (250g) cheddar cheese, shredded
- Salt and pepper to taste
- Optional salsa

Directions

- Cook the bacon until crisp in a 9- or 10-inch oven-proof skillet.
- Drain the bacon, saving some amount of the drippings.
- Heat the conserved drippings over medium-high heat.
- Asparagus, onion, and garlic should all be sautéed until the onion is tender.
- Set aside a third of the bacon crumbles.
- The remaining bacon, beaten eggs, parsley, seasoned salt, and pepper should all be combined in a large mixing basin.
- Swirl the egg mixture after adding it to the skillet.
- Top with the reserved bacon, tomato, and cheese.
- Cook, covered, over medium-low heat until the eggs are almost set, about 10 to 15 minutes.
- Preheat the broiler and position 6 inches from the flames was the skillet.
- Broil for a couple of minutes or until lightly browned.
- Please serve right away with optional salsa if you prefer.

14. OMELET SOUTHWESTERN

 5 minutes   15 minutes   4 servings

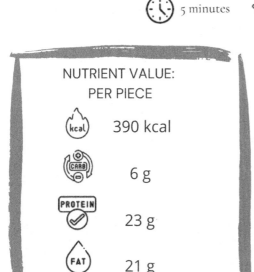

NUTRIENT VALUE:
PER PIECE

390 kcal

6 g

23 g

21 g

Ingredients

- 4.23 oz (120g) finely chopped onion
- 1 minced jalapeno pepper
- 1 tomato, sliced;
- sliced into 1-inch pieces, one avocado;
- 6 big eggs, softly beaten;
- 6 cooked and broken bacon pieces;
- 8.82 oz (250 g) Monterey Jack cheese;
- salt and pepper to the extent necessary
- Optional salsa

Directions

- Use a slotted spoon to remove the onion and jalapenos from the pan when they have softened in the oil in a big skillet and set them aside.
- The eggs should be cracked into the same skillet, covered, and cooked for 3–4 minutes at low heat.
- Add the bacon, tomato, avocado, onion combination and half a cup of cheese.
- Salt and pepper to the extent necessary
- On top of the filling, fold the omelet in half.
- Cook the eggs for 3 to 4 minutes or until they are done.
- To finish, include the remaining cheese.
- If you'd like, please top with salsa and serve.

15. STACK OF MASCARPONE-MUSHROOM FRITTATA

 25 minutes   20 minutes   6 servings

NUTRIENT VALUE:
PER PIECE

 468 kcal

 5 g

 20 g

 44 g

Ingredients

- 8 medium eggs
- 0.33 cups (80 ml) heavy whipping cream
- 4.23 oz (120g) grated Romano cheese
- 0.07 oz (3 g) teaspoon salt
- 2.54 fl oz (75 ml) olive oil, split
- 12 oz (340g) fresh mushrooms, cut
- 1 medium onion, cut in half and thinly sliced
- 1.06 oz (30g) fresh basil, minced
- 2 minced garlic cloves
- 0.04 oz (1g) black pepper
- 7.76 oz (220g) Mascarpone ricotta

- Whisk together the eggs, cream, 2.12 oz (60g) Romano cheese, and 0.11 oz (3g) salt in a large mixing dish.
- A 10-inch skillet with 1.01 fl oz (30 ml) of oil is heated to medium-high heat.
- The mushrooms and onion should be cooked and stirred until tender.
- After adding the basil, garlic, pepper, and remaining salt, cook and stir for an additional minute. Mascarpone and the remaining Romano cheese are added after being transferred to a mixing bowl.
- Heat 0.51 fl oz (15 ml) of oil in the same pan to medium-high heat.
- Include 150 ml or 5.07 fl oz of the egg mixture.
- At the edges, the mixture should quickly be set.
- Push cooked portions toward the center as the eggs set, allowing uncooked pieces to flow below.
- Allow to remain uncovered for 5-7 minutes or until fully set.
- Place on a serving tray, wrap with foil and maintain warm.
- Repeat with the remaining egg mixture to make two more frittatas, using the remaining oil as needed.
- Layer half of the mushroom mixture on top of one frittata on a serving plate.
- Layers should be repeated.
- Finish with the leftover frittata.

16. FRITTATA WITH ZUCCHINI AND GOUDA IN A SKILLET

 10 minutes   20 minutes   6 servings

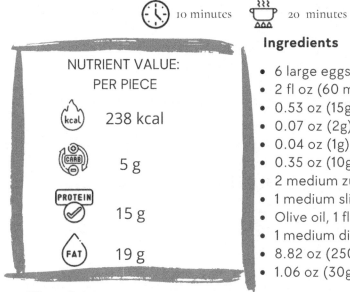

NUTRIENT VALUE:
PER PIECE

kcal   238 kcal

CARB   5 g

PROTEIN   15 g

FAT   19 g

Ingredients

- 6 large eggs
- 2 fl oz (60 ml) 2% milk
- 0.53 oz (15g) fresh oregano, diced
- 0.07 oz (2g) salt
- 0.04 oz (1g) black pepper
- 0.35 oz (10g) melted butter
- 2 medium zucchini, thinly sliced, 7.76 oz (220g) each
- 1 medium sliced onion
- Olive oil, 1 fluid ounce (30 ml)
- 1 medium diced tomato
- 8.82 oz (250g) Gouda cheese, shredded
- 1.06 oz (30g) fresh basil, minced

Directions

- Set aside the first five ingredients. Over medium heat, melt butter in a large nonstick pan.
- Combine with the onion and zucchini.
- Remove from the fire after cooking the veggies for 6 to 8 minutes or until tender.
- In the same skillet, heat the oil to medium-high heat. Mix in the egg mixture.
- Cook until the egg is set, gently raising the edges of the cooked egg to allow the liquid to run below.
- Serve with the zucchini mixture, diced tomato, and cheese on top.
- Cook for 2 to 3 minutes with the lid on or until the cheese is melted.
- Garnish with basil.

17. FLORENTINE EGG CASSEROLE

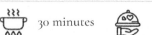 20 minutes   30 minutes   12 servings

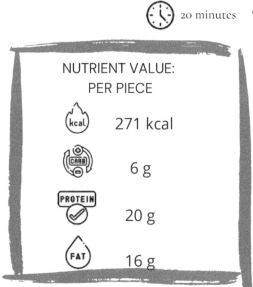

NUTRIENT VALUE:
PER PIECE

271 kcal

6 g

20 g

16 g

Ingredients

- 15.87 oz (450g) pork sausage in bulk
- 1.06 oz (30g) melted butter
- 1 big sliced onion
- 8.82 oz (250g) fresh sliced mushrooms
- 8.82 oz (250g) frozen chopped spinach, thawed and pressed dry
- 12 extra-large eggs
- 67.63 fl oz (2L) milk with 2% fat
- 8.82 oz (250g) Swiss cheese, shredded
- 8.82 oz (250g) sharp cheddar cheese, shredded
- 0.07 oz (2g) paprika

Directions

- Set the oven's temperature to 350°F (176°C).
- Sausage should be cooked 6 to 8 minutes over medium heat in a big pan and broken into crumbles. Once finished, drain and put in a 13 x 9-inch baking dish with butter.
- Melt butter over medium-high heat in the same skillet.
- Cook and stir the onion and mushrooms for 3 to 5 minutes or until soft.
- Add the spinach and stir. Over the meat, plate the vegetable mixture.
- Pour the egg mixture over the veggies after combining milk and eggs in a big mixing bowl.
- Add the cheese and paprika as garnish.
- Until the center is set and a thermometer placed into the center registers 160°F (73°C), bake for 30-35 minutes, uncovered.
- 10 minutes should pass before serving.

18. SCRAMBLED SPINACH–MUSHROOM EGGS

5 minutes   10 minutes   2 servings

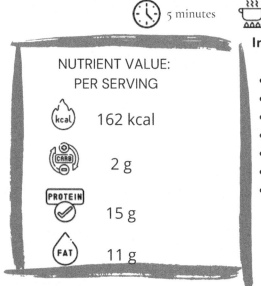

NUTRIENT VALUE:
PER SERVING

162 kcal

2 g

15 g

11 g

Ingredients

- Two big eggs and two big egg whites
- 0.04 oz (1g) pepper
- 0.04 oz (1g) salt
- 0.53 oz (15g) butter
- 4.23 oz (120g) fresh mushrooms, thinly sliced
- 4.23 oz (120g) chopped fresh baby spinach
- 1.06 oz (30g) provolone cheese, shredded

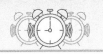

Directions

- In a small mixing dish, combine the eggs, egg whites, salt, and pepper.
- Melt the butter in a small nonstick pan over medium-high heat.
- The mushrooms should be tender after 3–4 minutes of cooking and stirring.
- Spinach is added and cooked while being constantly stirred.
- Medium-low heat should be used.
- Cook and whisk the egg mixture until there is no longer any liquid egg and the eggs have thickened.
- Add the cheese and stir.

19. QUICHE CUPS WITH BROCCOLI

🕐 10 minutes   🍲 15 minutes   🍽 6 servings

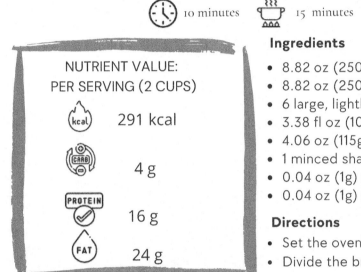

NUTRIENT VALUE:
PER SERVING (2 CUPS)

🔥 (kcal) 291 kcal

(CARB) 4 g

(PROTEIN) ✓ 16 g

(FAT) 24 g

Ingredients

- 8.82 oz (250g) fresh broccoli, chopped
- 8.82 oz (250g) pepper jack cheese, shredded
- 6 large, lightly beaten eggs
- 3.38 fl oz (100g) heavy whipping cream
- 4.06 oz (115g) bacon drippings
- 1 minced shallot
- 0.04 oz (1g) salt
- 0.04 oz (1g) pepper

Directions

- Set the oven's temperature to 350°F (176°C).
- Divide the broccoli and cheese among 12 muffin cups that have been oiled.
- Pour the remaining ingredients into the cups after whisking them together.
- Until the cheese has melted, bake for 15-20 minutes.

20. BREAKFAST CASSEROLE WITH GREEK FLAVORS

🕐 35 minutes   🍲 45 minutes   🍽 6 servings

NUTRIENT VALUE:
PER PIECE

🔥 (kcal) 179 kcal

(CARB) 7 g

(PROTEIN) ✓ 17 g

(FAT) 9 g

Ingredients

- 7.76 oz (220g) casing-free Italian turkey sausage links
- 4.23 oz (120g) green pepper, chopped
- 1 chopped shallot
- 8.82 oz (250g) rinsed, drained, and diced water-packed artichoke hearts
- 8.82 oz (250g) fresh broccoli, chopped
- 4.23 oz (120g) chopped sun-dried tomatoes (not packaged in oil)
- 6 big eggs
- 6 big egg whites

- 1.52 fl oz (45ml) fat-free milk
- 0.25 oz (7g) Italian seasoning
- 0.04 oz (1g) garlic powder
- 0.04 oz (1g) pepper
- 2.65 oz (75g) feta cheese, crumbled

Directions

- Set the oven's temperature to 350°F (176°C).
- Sausage, green pepper, and shallot should be cooked in a large pan over medium heat for 8 to 10 minutes or until the link is no longer pink. Drain.
- Pour the ingredients into an 8-inch square baking dish sprayed with cooking spray. Before serving, top with broccoli, artichokes, and sun-dried tomatoes.
- Combine eggs, egg whites, milk, and spices in a large mixing basin; pour over top.
- Add feta as a garnish.
- A knife in the middle should come clean after baking for 45 to 50 minutes with the top off.
- 10 minutes should pass before serving.

RECIPES
APPERITEZ
& SNACK

1. KABOBS WITH CHILLED CHICKEN AND CHEESE

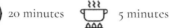 20 minutes 5 minutes 8 servings

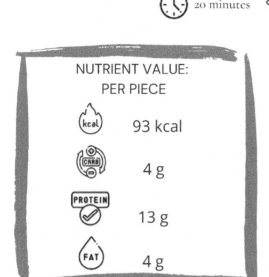

NUTRIENT VALUE:
PER PIECE

kcal — 93 kcal

CARB — 4 g

PROTEIN — 13 g

FAT — 4 g

Ingredients

- 2 g of salt
- 2 g chili powder
- 220 g boneless chicken breast
- 1 g pepper
- 15 ml balsamic vinegar
- 30 ml olive oil
- 140 g mozzarella cheese
- 16 cherry tomatoes

Directions

- Season the chicken cubes using salt, pepper, and cayenne.
- Pour into a large mixing basin.
- Add the vinegar and toss to coat.
- Covered, chill for three to four hours.
- After draining the chicken, save the marinade.
- In a big skillet, heat the oil over medium heat.
- Cook the chicken till the meat is no longer pinkish.
- Allow to cool slightly—thread chicken, cheese, and tomatoes onto wooden skewers in alternate directions. Serve chilled.

2. DEVILED EGGS WITH BACON AND CHEDDAR

 10 minutes 20 minutes 10 servings

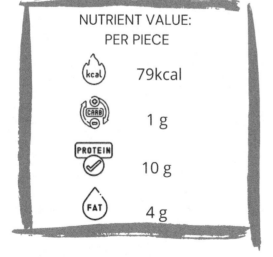

NUTRIENT VALUE:
PER PIECE

kcal — 79kcal

CARB — 1 g

PROTEIN — 10 g

FAT — 4 g

Ingredients

- 12 big hard-boiled eggs
- 110 g mayonnaise
- 4 cooked bacon strips
- 30 g cheddar cheese
- 15 ml mustard honey
- 1 g pepper

Directions

- Split the eggs lengthwise, scoop off the yolks, and save the whites.
- In a little basin, mash the yolks.
- Add the mayonnaise, bacon, cheese, mustard, and pepper to a mixing dish.
- Fill egg whites with stuffing or pipe with a pastry bag.
- Refrigerate until ready to serve.

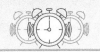
3. LIME WITH SPICED HOT CHIPOTLE SPINACH AND ARTICHOKE DIP

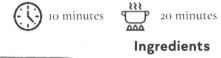 10 minutes   20 minutes   4 servings

NUTRIENT VALUE:
PER SERVING

 164 kcal

 3 g

 7 g

 14 g

Ingredients

- 1 lb (450g) mozzarella cheese, shredded
- 8 oz (220g) softened cream cheese
- 4 oz (120g) mayonnaise
- 4 oz (120g) Parmesan cheese, grated
- 2 finely chopped chipotle chiles in adobo sauce
- 1/4 cup (60ml) lime juice
- 1 tablespoon (15ml) grated lime zest
- 1/4 teaspoon (1g) kosher salt
- 1/4 teaspoon (1g) pepper
- 14 oz (400g) drained and finely chopped water-packed artichoke hearts
- 12 oz (350g) frozen chopped spinach, thawed and pressed dry
- 1 large garlic clove, finely chopped
- 3 green onions, chopped
- Baked pita chips, tortilla chips, sliced French bread baguettes, or different crackers are optional.

Directions

- Preheat the oven to 400°F.
- Combine the mozzarella cheese, cream cheese, mayonnaise, and 2 oz grated Parmesan cheese in a mixing bowl.
- Mix in the following 9 components.
- Add the remaining Parmesan on top before pouring it into a deep dish pie plate.
- Bake for 20 to 25 minutes, till bubbling and golden brown.
- As preferred, serve with crackers, baguette slices, pita, or tortilla chips.

4. MINIATURE FRITTATAS DE SPINACH

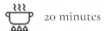 10 minutes   20 minutes   8 servings

NUTRIENT VALUE:
PER PIECE

128 kcal

4 g

10 g

9 g

Ingredients

- 1 cup (250 g) ricotta cheese (whole milk)
- 1/2 teaspoon (2 g) dried oregano
- 1 cup (100 g) grated Parmesan cheese
- 1/2 cup (75 g) chopped fresh mushrooms
- 1/4 teaspoon (1 g) pepper
- 1 box frozen chopped spinach (10oz - 220 g), thawed and pressed dry
- 1 large egg
- 1/4 teaspoon (1 g) salt

Directions

- The oven should be heated to 390°F (200°C).
- In a small dish, mix all ingredients.
- The cheese mixture should be poured into every one of the 24 buttered mini-muffin tins to a height of three-quarters.
- Until the center is completely set, bake the cake for 20 to 25 minutes.
- To loosen frittatas, carefully run a knife over the sides of the muffin cups.
- Serve hot.

5. CRAB AVOCADO BOATS

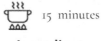 5 minutes 15 minutes 8 servings

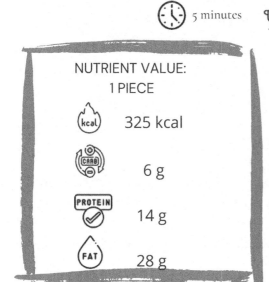

NUTRIENT VALUE:
1 PIECE

kcal   325 kcal

CARB   6 g

PROTEIN   14 g

FAT   28 g

Ingredients

- 5 peeled and halved medium-ripe avocados
- 1/2 cup (120 g) mayonnaise
- 2 tablespoons (30 ml) lemon juice
- 2 cans (6 ounces each - 170 g) of drained lump crabmeat
- 1/2 cup (60 g) fresh cilantro, chopped
- 2 tablespoons (30 g) finely minced chives
- 1 seeded and minced serrano pepper
- 1 tablespoon (15 g) drained capers
- 1/4 teaspoon (1 g) pepper
- 2 cups (250 g) pepper jack cheese, shredded
- 1/4 teaspoon (2 g) paprika
- slices of lemon

Directions

- Preheat the oven to 350°F (175°C).
- Scoop out some flesh from each avocado half to create a hollow space for the filling. Place the hollowed avocado halves in a baking dish.
- In a bowl, mix the mayonnaise and lemon juice until well combined.
- Add the drained lump crabmeat, chopped cilantro, chives, serrano pepper, drained capers, and pepper to the mayonnaise mixture. Stir everything together until evenly mixed.
- Spoon the crab mixture into each avocado half, filling them generously.
- Sprinkle the shredded pepper jack cheese on top of the crab-filled avocados.
- Dust the tops with paprika for added flavor and color.
- Bake the avocado boats in the oven for 10-15 minutes, or until the cheese is melted and bubbly and the avocados are warmed.
- Remove from the oven and let them cool slightly.
- Garnish each boat with a slice of lemon.

6. KABOBS FROM A GREEK DELI

 240 minutes 0 minutes 10 servings

Ingredients

- 1 lb (450 g) part-skim mozzarella cheese, cubed
- 24 florets of fresh broccoli (about 10 ounces)
- 1/2 cup (120 g) vinaigrette (Greek)
- 24 firm salami slices
- 2 jars (7 ounces each -200 g) delicious red peppers, roasted, drained, and sliced into 24 strips

Directions

- Mix the cheese, broccoli, and vinaigrette in a shallow bowl.
- For four hours, cover and chill.
- Drain the cheese and broccoli while retaining the vinaigrette.

NUTRIENT VALUE:
PER PIECE

 109 kcal

 2 g

 9 g

 7 g

- Thread cheese, salami, broccoli, and peppers alternately on 24 appetizer skewers.
- Drizzle with the reserved vinaigrette.

7. WRAPPED CALIFORNIA BURGERS

 30 minutes 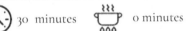 0 minutes 4 servings

Ingredients

- 2 tablespoons (30 g) of Miracle Whip Light
- 1 lb (450 g) ground beef, lean
- 1/2 teaspoon (2 g) of salt
- 1/4 cup (75 g) red onion, chopped
- 1/4 teaspoon (1 g) pepper
- 8 leaves Bibb lettuce
- 1/4 cup (75 g) feta cheese, crumbled
- 1/2 ripe medium avocado
- Optional: chopped cherry tomatoes

Directions

- Combine the meat with salt, pepper, and chopped onion. Toss gently but thoroughly.

NUTRIENT VALUE:
2 PIECES

 252 kcal

 5 g

 24 g

 15 g

- Make eight patties that are 1/2 inch thick.
- The burgers should be broiler-grilled or covered-grilled for 3–4 minutes on both sides till an instant-read thermometer registers 160°.
- Sandwich the patties between lettuce leaves.
- Spread feta and Miracle Whip on top of the burgers.
- Top with avocado, and tomatoes, if desired.

8. CHICKEN TEX–MEX STRIPS

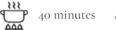 20 minutes 40 minutes 4 servings

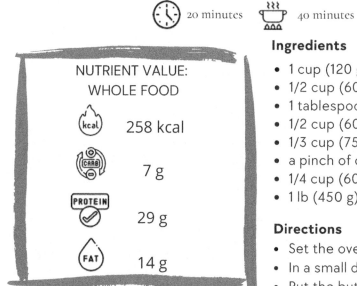

NUTRIENT VALUE:
WHOLE FOOD

258 kcal

7 g

29 g

14 g

Ingredients

- 1 cup (120 g) corn chips, finely crushed
- 1/2 cup (60 g) panko bread crumbs
- 1 tablespoon (15 g) dry bread crumbs
- 1/2 cup (60 g) Mexican cheese blend, finely shredded
- 1/3 cup (75 g) taco seasoning
- a pinch of cayenne pepper
- 1/4 cup (60 g) melted butter
- 1 lb (450 g) tenderloins of chicken

Directions

- Set the oven to 400°F
- In a small dish, mix the first six ingredients.
- Put the butter in a different, small bowl.

- The chicken is first dipped in butter, then rolled through the crumb mix and pressed to adhere. A foiled baking pan measuring 15 by 10 by 1 inch should contain the chicken.
- Bake for 15 minutes, turning the pan halfway through, till a thermometer poked into the chicken registers 165°.

9. GUACAMOLE WITH CAJUN SHRIMP AND RED PEPPER

 15 minutes 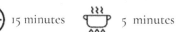 5 minutes 6 servings

NUTRIENT VALUE:
PER SERVING

 152 kcal

 5 g

 9 g

 11 g

Ingredients

- 3 medium ripe avocados, peeled and cubed
- 3 tablespoons (45 ml) fresh lime juice
- 1 teaspoon (5 g) kosher salt
- Cajun Shrimp (8 oz or 220 g)
- 1/2 cup (60 g) sweet red pepper, chopped

Directions

- Peel and cube 3 medium-ripe avocados.
- In a bowl, combine the avocado cubes with 3 tablespoons (45 ml) of fresh lime juice.
- Sprinkle 1 teaspoon (5 g) of kosher salt over the avocado mixture and gently toss to coat.

- Prepare Cajun shrimp by cooking 8 oz (220 g) of shrimp with Cajun seasoning according to your preferred method (grilling, sautéing, etc.).
- Chop 1/2 cup (60 g) of sweet red pepper.
- Once the shrimp is cooked, let it cool slightly, and then add it to the avocado mixture.
- Mix in the chopped sweet red pepper.

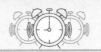
- Season with 1/4 teaspoon (1 g) of salt or to taste.
- Add 1/4 cup (60 ml) of water to the skillet and stir to deglaze the pan.
- Mix in 1 tablespoon (15 g) of Dijon mustard, ensuring the onions are coated.
- Add 1 lb (450 g) of thinly sliced Brussels sprouts to the skillet and toss them in the onion mixture.
- Cook the Brussels sprouts until tender and slightly browned, about 5-7 minutes.
- Drizzle 1 tablespoon (15 ml) of cider vinegar over the Brussels sprouts and stir to combine.
- Sprinkle the crumbled bacon on top of the dish before serving.

10. BEST BAKED POTATO

 10 minutes 60 minutes 2 servings

NUTRIENT VALUE:
PER RECIPE

 284 kcal

 30 g

 20 g

 1 g

Ingredients

- 1 big russet potato
- 1 tablespoon (15 ml) canola oil
- kosher salt (to taste)

Directions

- Preheat the oven to 425°F (218°C).
- Wash and scrub the russet potato to remove any dirt.
- You can cut the potato into thin strips or wedges, depending on what you prefer.
- In a large bowl, toss the potato strips with 1 tablespoon (15 ml) of canola oil, ensuring they are coated evenly.
- Spread the potatoes in a single layer on a baking sheet lined with parchment paper.
- Sprinkle kosher salt over the potatoes, adjusting the amount to taste.
- Bake the potatoes in the oven for about 25-30 minutes or until golden brown and crispy.
- Remove the potatoes from the oven and let them cool slightly before serving.

11. ROASTED BROCCOLI

 5 minutes 20 minutes 4 servings

Ingredients

- 4 cups broccoli florets
- 1 tbsp. olive oil
- Salt and pepper to taste

Directions

- Preheat your oven to 400°F
- Add broccoli in a zip bag alongside oil and shake until coated

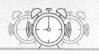
NUTRIENT VALUE:
PER SERVING

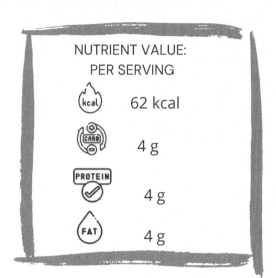

kcal — 62 kcal

CARB — 4 g

PROTEIN — 4 g

FAT — 4 g

- Add seasoning and shake again
- Spread the broccoli out on the baking sheet, and bake for 20 minutes
- Let it cool and serve.

12. ALMOND FLOUR MUFFINS

 15 minutes 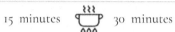 30 minutes 8 servings

Ingredients

NUTRIENT VALUE:
PER RECIPE

kcal — 130 kcal

CARB — 1 g

PROTEIN — 2 g

FAT — 5 g

- ⅓ cup pumpkin puree
- 3 eggs
- 2 tbsps. agave nectar
- 2 tbsps. coconut oil
- 1 tsp. vanilla extract
- 1 tsp. white vinegar
- 1 cup chopped fruits
- 1 tsp. baking soda
- ½ tsp. salt

Directions

- Preheat the oven to 350°F.
- Line the muffin tin with paper liners
- In the first mixing bowl, whisk the almond flour, salt, and baking soda.
- In the second mixing bowl, whisk the pumpkin puree, eggs, coconut oil, agave nectar, vanilla extract, and vinegar.
- Now add this puree mix from the second bowl to the first bowl and blend everything well.
- Add the chopped fruits to the blend.
- Pour the mixture into the muffin cups in your pan.
- Bake for 15-20 minutes. Ensure that the contents have been set in the center, and a golden-brown lining has started to appear at the edges.
- Transfer the muffins to a cooling rack and let them cool completely.

RECIPES
PASTA

1. PASTA WITH CREAMY SALMON

 5 minutes 15 minutes 3 servings

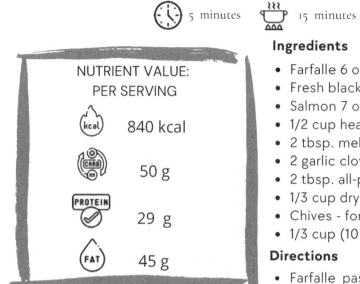

NUTRIENT VALUE:
PER SERVING

kcal — 840 kcal

CARB — 50 g

PROTEIN — 29 g

FAT — 45 g

Ingredients

- Farfalle 6 ounces (170 g)
- Fresh black pepper and sea salt (to taste)
- Salmon 7 ounces salmon (200 g)
- 1/2 cup heavy cream (120 g) heavy cream
- 2 tbsp. melted butter (30 g)
- 2 garlic cloves
- 2 tbsp. all-purpose flour (10 g)
- 1/3 cup dry white wine (100 ml)
- Chives - for decoration
- 1/3 cup (100 ml) turkey stock

Directions

- Farfalle pasta needs to be cooked according to the instructions on the package. Drain, then set apart.
- On, warm up the melted butter in the pan. When the salmon is cooked thoroughly, you can cook it in the pan. The salmon should be taken out of the pan and placed aside.
- The minced garlic should be sauteed in the same pan for about a minute until it smells aromatic.
- After mixing, add the all-purpose flour, then cook for another minute.
- It is necessary to blend white wine and turkey stock before simmering the mixture till it barely thickens.
- As the heat is reduced, stir in the heavy cream. After cooking for a few minutes, the sauce will start to thicken.
- After cooking the fish, flake it into the sauce and season it with sea salt and black pepper.
- Cooked farfalle pasta has to be blended with the sauce and poured into it before serving.
- With a garnish of chives, serve the farfalle with creamy salmon.

2. SQUASH CASSEROLE WITH TURKEY SPAGHETTI

 25 minutes 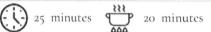 20 minutes 8 servings

Ingredients

- 5 tbsp. (75 g) butter
- 2 cups (450 g) cooked turkey
- 1 cup (250 g) celery
- 1 moderate onion
- 1 poblano pepper - 1 pinch of cumin
- 1/2 cup (100 ml) turkey broth
- A pinch of black pepper
- 1 bell pepper - 2 pinches of garlic powder
- 3 cups (350 g) Colby Jack cheese
- 5 garlic cloves

- 1 cup (250 g) green chilies and
- 1 spaghetti squash (about 2 pounds)
- 1 can of tomatoes
- 4 cups (1 liter) heavy cream
- 4 ounces (120 g) cream cheese

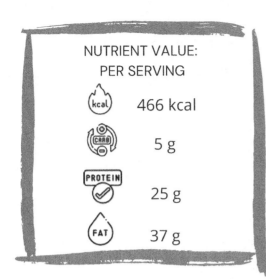

NUTRIENT VALUE:
PER SERVING

466 kcal

5 g

25 g

37 g

Directions

- Adjust the oven's thermostat to 400°F (200°C). After scooping out the seeds, split the spaghetti squash into halves lengthwise, and arrange the pieces on a baking sheet. Add melted butter to the sides. For about 40 minutes, roast the squash in the oven till it is soft and readily shreds with a fork. The spaghetti squash should now be left aside.
- Inside a pan, melt the butter. Add the chopped celery, bell pepper, onion, and poblano pepper. The vegetables should be cooked till soft.
- Once the garlic is aromatic, stir it and simmer for another minute.
- Add the chopped canned tomatoes, green chilies, and the turkey broth. A few minutes of simmering should be enough to thicken the liquid slightly.
- Heating the heavy cream on a low flame in a separate pan. Black pepper, cumin, garlic powder, and cream cheese should all be added. Stirring will smooth out the sauce and melt the cream cheese.
- Cooked turkey, sautéed veggies, and creamy sauce should all be mixed in the pan. Mix thoroughly.
- In a baking dish, arrange half of the spaghetti squash strands. Add half of the turkey and vegetable cream mixture on top. Add half of the Colby Jack cheese that has been chopped.
- Repeat the layering With the remaining spaghetti squash, creamy turkey mixture, and cheese.
- Bake at 375°F (190°C) in a set-up oven for approximately twenty-five to thirty minutes till the cheese is melted and bubbling.
- Serve the creamy turkey spaghetti squash bake hot, and enjoy!

3. KETO LASAGNA

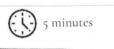 5 minutes   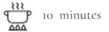 10 minutes   4 servings

NUTRIENT VALUE:
PER RECIPE

130 kcal

1 g

2 g

5 g

Ingredients

- 1 cup (250 g) Parmesan cheese
- 2 pinches of Italian seasoning
- Low-carb marinara sauce
- A pinch of black pepper
- 2 cups (250 g) mozzarella cheese
- 1 pound (450 g) sausage
- 4 garlic cloves
- 1 cup (250 g) ricotta cheese
- 1 pinch of salt

Directions

- Your oven should be set at 375°F (190°C).
- Cook the sausage in a pan till it is well-cooked and browned. Remove any extra fat.
- The marinara sauce should be added and cooked thoroughly after a few minutes of simmering.

- Combine the mozzarella and ricotta with half of the Parmesan in a bowl.
- Add salt, black pepper, chopped garlic, and Italian seasoning to the cheese mixture.
- In a baking dish, distribute half the sausage with the sauce mixture on the bottom.
- The link is topped with half of the cheese mixture.
- Repeat the process with the other ingredients, layering the cheese mixture first, then the sausage and sauce.
- Top with the remaining Parmesan cheese.
- Bake for about twenty-five minutes in the preheated oven.
- Before serving, allow it cool for a while.

4. KETO MUSHROOM PASTA

 20 minutes   40 minutes   4 servings

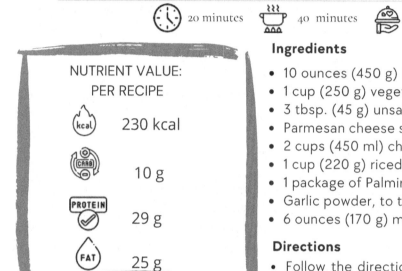

NUTRIENT VALUE:
PER RECIPE

230 kcal

10 g

29 g

25 g

Ingredients

- 10 ounces (450 g) fresh baby spinach
- 1 cup (250 g) vegetable stock
- 3 tbsp. (45 g) unsalted butter
- Parmesan cheese seasoned with salt and pepper
- 2 cups (450 ml) choice of milk
- 1 cup (220 g) riced cauliflower
- 1 package of Palmini palm hearts linguini
- Garlic powder, to taste
- 6 ounces (170 g) mushrooms

Directions

- Follow the directions on the package for preparing the Palmini palm hearts linguine. Drain, then set apart.
- Butter should be melted inside a pan.
- The mushrooms should now be added to the pan and cooked till tender and just starting to brown.
- Fresh baby spinach is added and cooked till wilted.
- Riced cauliflower should be added to the pan and cooked for a few minutes till soft.
- Add the vegetable stock, and then boil the mixture.
- For more flavor, add a bit additional garlic powder.
- As the sauce thickens, turn down the heat and gradually mix in the desired milk.
- Once the sauce has reached the desired consistency, add the cooked Palmini linguini to the pan.
- Toss everything together till the linguini is evenly coated with the creamy vegetable sauce.
- Please make sure to serve the linguini hot and, if you'd like, top with Parmesan cheese seasoned with salt and pepper for extra flavor.

5. BLUE CHEESE ZOODLES

 5 minutes   12 minutes   4 servings

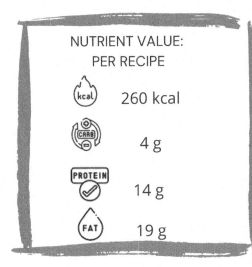

NUTRIENT VALUE:
PER RECIPE

260 kcal

4 g

14 g

19 g

Ingredients

- 2 tbsp. (30 ml) extra-virgin olive oil
- 2 minced garlic cloves
- 6 slices of bacon
- 2 fresh basil leaves, cut into thin strips
- 1 tomato
- 1 cup (120 g) blue cheese crumbles
- 2 pounds (1 kg) of zoodles (zucchini noodles)

Directions

- Cook the bacon till it is crispy in a pan. Then take it out and place it aside.
- Add the extra virgin olive oil and minced garlic to the same pan. Garlic should be sautéed till it smells good and starts to become golden.
- Now put the tomatoes in the pan and let them cook for a minute.
- When zucchini noodles are cooked through and soft but still have a slight crunch, put them in the pan and simmer for a few minutes.
- Crumble the cooked bacon on the zoodles in the pan.
- Garnish the blue cheese crumbles o zoodles and bacon.
- Stir everything together gently, allowing the blue cheese to melt slightly, and coat the zoodles.
- Garnish with the cut basil leaves for fresh flavor and aroma.

6. LASAGNA WITH ZUCCHINI

 20 minutes 45 minutes 8 servings

NUTRIENT VALUE:
PER RECIPE

333 kcal

2 g

13 g

25 g

Ingredients

- 2 pinches of (3 g) Italian seasoning
- 1 tbsp. (10 ml) olive oil
- 1/3 cup (75 g) parmesan cheese
- 9 ounces (250 g) mozzarella cheese
- 2 pinches of (3 g) salt
- 1 pinch of (2 g) black pepper
- 1/3 cup (75 g) ricotta cheese
- 1 zucchini
- A pinch of (1 g) anise seeds
- 1 1/2 cups (350 ml) marinara sauce
- 2 pinches of (3 g) garlic powder
- 1 pound (450 g) beef
- 1 egg

Directions

- The oven temperature must be set at 375°F (190°C).
- Remove the seeds after slicing the zucchini (courgette) in half lengthwise.
- Olive oil should be heated in a pan over a medium flame. When the meat is added, crumble it as it cooks till it is browned. Add anise seeds, Italian seasoning, salt, and pepper for seasoning.
- Add marinara sauce, then simmer for a few minutes to combine the flavors.
- Combine the ricotta, parmesan, and egg with garlic powder in a separate bowl.

- The meat mixture should be spooned into each side of the zucchini, followed by the ricotta cheese mixture.
- Place the stuffed zucchini halves in a baking dish and con each one with fresh mozzarella cheese.
- Bake for about twenty-five minutes, till zucchini becomes tender and the cheese is melted and bubbly.
- Garnish with some additional herbs or parmesan cheese if desired, and serve the delicious and comforting stuffed zucchini hot!

7. CREAMY KETO PUMPKIN ALFREDO

 10 minutes 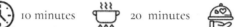 20 minutes 6 servings

NUTRIENT VALUE:
PER RECIPE

kcal   218 kcal

CARB   6 g

PROTEIN   5 g

FAT   8 g

Ingredients

- 2 tbsp. (30 g) melted butter
- 3 pounds (1.5 kg) of zoodles (zucchini noodles)
- A pinch of (1 g) black pepper
- 1 cup (120 g) parmesan cheese
- A pinch of (1 g) nutmeg
- 4 cups (1 kg) heavy cream
- 1 pinch of (2 g) salt
- 1 cup (250 g) pureed pumpkin
- 2 garlic cloves

Directions

- Saute garlic in melted butter for a minute.
- Cook for one more minute after stirring in the pumpkin puree.
- Heavy cream should be added once the mixture has a mild boil. Give it a few minutes to simmer so that the flavors may mingle.
- Salt, nutmeg, and black pepper are used to season the sauce. To suit your preferences, you can adjust the seasoning.
- Parmesan cheese is added, and the sauce is simmered until it slightly thickens.
- Boil zoodles till they are soft but still have a slight crunch.
- Drain the zoodles and add them to the pumpkin cream sauce. Toss everything together till the zoodles are well coated with creamy goodness.
- You can serve the pumpkin cream zoodles hot, garnished with additional parmesan cheese and a sprinkle of fresh herbs if you'd like.

8. ALFREDO CREAMY KETO GARLIC AND OLIVE PASTA

 5 minutes 15 minutes 6 servings

Ingredients

- 2 teaspoons (10 g) Melted butter
- Salt & pepper: to taste
- 3.3 pounds (1.5 kg) of zucchini noodles
- 1 egg yolk
- 8.8 ounces (250 g) Parmesan cheese
- 2 cloves Minced garlic cloves
- 8.8 ounces (250 g) Chopped green olives
- 1.5 liters Thick cream

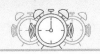
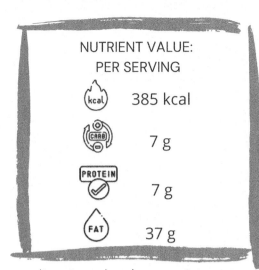

NUTRIENT VALUE:
PER SERVING

kcal 385 kcal

CARB 7 g

PROTEIN 7 g

FAT 37 g

Directions

- In a large skillet, melt the butter over medium heat.
- Season the melted butter with salt and pepper according to your taste preferences.
- Add the zoodles (zucchini noodles) to the skillet and sauté them until they are tender-crisp. This may take about 3-5 minutes.
- In a separate bowl, whisk the egg yolk until it is well beaten.
- Gradually add the grated Parmesan cheese to the beaten egg yolk, stirring constantly to create a smooth mixture.
- Stir in the minced garlic cloves and chopped green olives into the cheese mixture.
- Lower the heat of the skillet and pour the thick cream into the zoodles. Stir well to combine.
- Add the prepared cheese, egg, garlic, and olive mixture to the zoodles and cream in the skillet. Toss everything together until the zoodles are well coated with creamy sauce.
- Continue to cook the zoodles and sauce for a few more minutes, allowing the flavors to meld and the sauce to thicken slightly.
- Remove the skillet from the heat and serve the creamy zoodles immediately. Garnish with extra Parmesan cheese, if desired.

9. KETO FETA BAKED PASTA

 20 minutes   35 minutes   4 servings

NUTRIENT VALUE:
PER RECIPE

kcal 343 kcal

CARB 3 g

PROTEIN 14 g

FAT 26 g

Ingredients

- 1/2 cup (120 ml) extra-virgin olive oil
- 7 ounces (190 g) hearts of palm or zucchini noodles
- 2 garlic cloves
- 1 pinch of (3 g) sea salt
- 7 ounces (200 g) of feta cheese
- 3 fresh basil leaves
- 1 cup (450 g) Kalamata olives
- 1/2 pound (250 g) turkey
- 4 pounds (2 kg) grape tomatoes

Directions

- Your oven should be set at 400°F (204°C).
- The grape tomatoes should be arranged in a single layer on a baking pan.
- To uniformly coat the tomatoes, sprinkle the tomatoes with the minced garlic, add the extra virgin olive oil, then mix everything.
- The tomatoes should be roasted in the preheated oven for a total of twenty minutes or till they begin to burst and exude juices.
- While roasting tomatoes, crumble the feta cheese into pieces and chop the fresh basil leaves.
- Once the tomatoes are roasted, take them out and let them cool down.

- In a dish, mix the roasted tomatoes with the Kalamata olives, turkey, and chopped hearts of palm or zucchini noodles.
- Season the salad with sea salt and gently toss everything together to mix.
- Sprinkle the crumbled feta cheese and chopped basil on the salad and give it one final toss to incorporate all the flavors.
- Serve the Mediterranean-inspired salad, either warm or chilled.

10. NOODLES WITH ZUCCHINI

10 minutes   6 minutes   10 servings

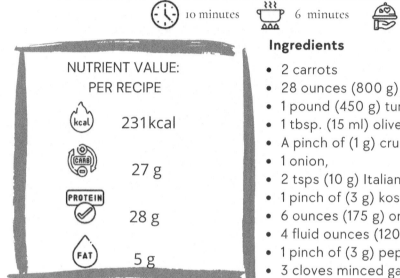

NUTRIENT VALUE:
PER RECIPE

231kcal

27 g

28 g

5 g

Ingredients

- 2 carrots
- 28 ounces (800 g) of organic tomato puree
- 1 pound (450 g) turkey
- 1 tbsp. (15 ml) olive oil
- A pinch of (1 g) crushed red pepper flakes
- 1 onion,
- 2 tsps (10 g) Italian herb blend
- 1 pinch of (3 g) kosher salt
- 6 ounces (175 g) organic can of tomato paste
- 4 fluid ounces (120 ml) of turkey stock
- 1 pinch of (3 g) pepper
- 3 cloves minced garlic

To make zucchini noodles
- 3–6 moderate zucchini

Directions:
- Olive oil should be heated over in a pan or saucepan.
- To the saucepan, add the minced onions and garlic.
- Cook the turkey in the saucepan after adding it till it is well browned.
- The carrots should soften after you stir them in and simmer for a few minutes. Add the tomato paste and puree made from organic tomatoes. Stir to combine.
- Add the crushed red pepper flakes, kosher salt, pepper, Italian herb mix, and turkey stock. Stir everything till it is well combined.
- Allow the sauce to simmer for twenty minutes on low heat so the flavors can mingle and the sauce may thicken.
- When adjusting the seasoning, taste the sauce and add salt or pepper as desired.
- The sauce is prepared for serving after it has reached the required thickness.

11. SHRIMP ROASTED IN GARLIC WITH ZUCCHINI PASTA

 10 minutes   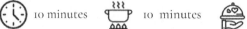 10 minutes   2 servings

Ingredients

- 0.35 ounces (10 g) melted ghee (or olive oil)
- 2 moderate zucchini
- 2 cloves minced garlic
- 0.04 ounces (1 g) salt
- 2 tsps (10 ml) olive oil
- Fresh pepper to taste
- 8.8 ounces (250 g) frozen shrimp
- 1 lemon, zested and juiced

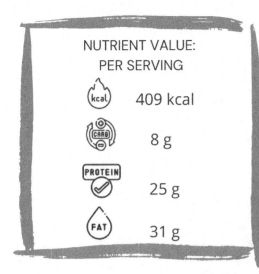

NUTRIENT VALUE:
PER SERVING

409 kcal

8 g

25 g

31 g

Directions

- Thaw the frozen shrimp according to the package instructions.
- Olive oil should be heated in a pan over a medium-high flame.
- Garlic that has been minced should be added to the pan and then sautéed till fragrant.
- Spread out the defrosted shrimp in one layer in the pan.
- Now add salt along with fresh pepper while preparing the shrimp.
- Then pour the melted ghee into the pan after lowering the heat to low. To uniformly coat the shrimp, mix everything.
- Lemon zest should be added to the pan with the shrimp after been zested and added.
- Lemon juice should be squeezed over the shrimp to impart a tart citrus taste.
- While the shrimp is finishing cooking, prepare the zucchini. Use a spiralizer or a vegetable peeler to create zucchini noodles (zoodles).
- Add the zucchini noodles to the pan with the shrimp, tossing them together until the zoodles are heated and slightly softened.
- Serve the flavorful shrimp and zucchini noodles immediately, and enjoy a light and delicious low-carb meal packed with protein and nutrients.

12. PESTO ZUCCHINI PASTA

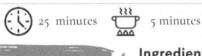 25 minutes 5 minutes 4 servings

NUTRIENT VALUE:
PER SERVING

220 kcal

9 g

4 g

20 g

Ingredients

- 8.8 ounces (250 g) cherry tomatoes
- 2 zucchini (seasoned with salt)

For the pesto:

- 2 pinches of (5 ml) lemon juice
- 3.5 ounces (100 g) toasted walnuts
- 1 roasted garlic head
- 2.5 fluid ounces (75 ml) of extra virgin olive oil
- 15.8 ounces (450 g) fresh basil leaves, plus a couple for garnish

Directions

- The oven should be set to 400°F (200°C).
- Slice the zucchini into thin pieces and sprinkle with salt.
- Bake the zucchini slices in the oven for ten minutes.
- Make the pesto while the zucchini finishes roasting. Combine the walnuts, garlic cloves, fresh basil leaves, and lemon juice in a food processor.
- Use the food processor to pulse the items until they are finely minced while adding the oil.
- ·When your zucchini slices are done, take them out of the oven and give them a little moment to cool.
- Slices of roasted zucchini and cherry tomatoes should be combined in a bowl.

- When the zucchini and tomatoes are all covered in the tasty pesto, put the prepared pesto in the bowl, then stir everything together.
- Garnish the meal with a few basil leaves for a splash of color and freshness.

13. SPAGHETTI WITH MEATBALLS (LOW CARB SPAGHETTI)

10 minutes   30 minutes   4 servings

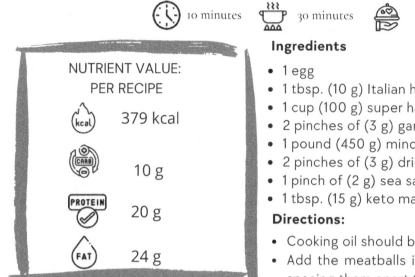

NUTRIENT VALUE:
PER RECIPE

kcal   379 kcal

CARB   10 g

PROTEIN   20 g

FAT   24 g

Ingredients

- 1 egg
- 1 tbsp. (10 g) Italian herb mixture
- 1 cup (100 g) super hazelnut flour
- 2 pinches of (3 g) garlic powder
- 1 pound (450 g) minced beef
- 2 pinches of (3 g) dried oregano
- 1 pinch of (2 g) sea salt
- 1 tbsp. (15 g) keto marinara sauce

Directions:

- Cooking oil should be heated in a frying pan.
- Add the meatballs into the pan once the oil is heated, spacing them apart to ensure uniform cooking.
- The meatballs should be fried on each side for 3–4 minutes or until well cooked.
- Mix the minced beef, hazelnut flour, Italian herb mixture, dried oregano, garlic powder, and sea salt in a mixing bowl.
- Crack the egg into the bowl with the other ingredients.
- Using clean hands, mix all the ingredients till well mixed. Ensure that the egg and seasonings are evenly distributed throughout the beef mixture.
- Form the mixture into meatballs of your desired size. You can make them for bite-sized snacks or r for a hearty meal.
- While the meatballs are cooking, warm the keto marinara sauce in a pan or microwave.
- When the meatballs are done, transfer them to a serving dish and drizzle the warm keto marinara sauce on them.

14. PASTA CREAMY PESTO RUTABAGA

5 minutes   10 minutes   3 servings

Ingredients

- 2 tbsp. (30 g) minced red onion
- 1/2 cup (100 g) grape tomatoes,
- 2 pinches of (5 ml) avocado, coconut, or olive oil
- 1-2 rutabagas noodles (3 cups of noodles) hazelnut milk

- Crushed red pepper, to taste
- 1/3 cup (100 ml) unsweetened Hazelnut Breeze
- 2 tbsp. (30 g) prepared pesto

Directions:

- Heat oil first in a pan, then add the red onion after mincing it to the pan and sauté until it becomes fragrant and slightly translucent.
- Add the spiralized rutabaga noodles to the pan. Toss them in the oil and onions, allowing

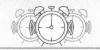
them to cook until they are tender-crisp.

- Pour the unsweetened Hazelnut Breeze hazelnut milk on the noodles. The milk will add creaminess and a subtle nutty flavor to the dish.
- Stir in the prepared pesto, coating the noodles and vegetables with its delicious herbal aroma.
- If you desire some heat, sprinkle crushed red pepper on the noodles to add a kick of spice.
- Lastly, add the grape tomatoes to the pan. They will provide bursts of juicy sweetness and a pop of vibrant color to the dish.
- I was cooking and tossing the ingredients until everything was heated through and well mixed.
- Remove the pan from the heat once the rutabaga noodles are cooked to your preferred texture and the flavors have melded.

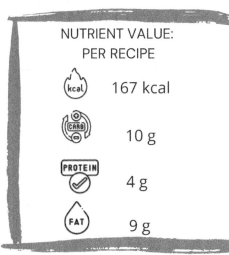

NUTRIENT VALUE:
PER RECIPE

167 kcal

10 g

4 g

9 g

15. ASPARAGUS POWDERS WITH LOW CARB

 10 minutes 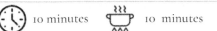 10 minutes 4 servings

NUTRIENT VALUE:
PER RECIPE

169 kcal

0 g

3 g

5 g

Ingredients

- 2 tbsp. (30 ml) lemon juice and 2 pinches of (3 ml) lemon zest cut into noodles
- 1 tbsp. (15 g) melted butter
- 4 cups (1 liter) heavy cream
- 2 garlic cloves, smashed
- 1/4 cup (30 g) Parmesan cheese
- 2 pinches of (3 g) Dijon mustard
- 1 pound (450 g) asparagus

Directions:

- Heat the melted butter in a pan or pot on moderate heat.
- Add the asparagus noodles to the pan and sauté them in the butter till they become tender-crisp.
- Pour the thick cream into the pan, allowing it to coat the asparagus noodles.
- It is time to add lemon juice and, lemon zest, dijon mustard to the pan.
- You may impart their fragrant flavor to the sauce by smashing the garlic cloves.
- Sprinkle some Parmesan cheese over the sauce.
- As the flavors converge and the sauce thickens, cook the sauce and the asparagus noodles together.
- Remove the pan from the heat Once the asparagus noodles are cooked to your desired tenderness and the sauce has reached your preferred consistency.

16. BUTTERNUT SQUASH RISOTTO

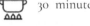 10 minutes 30 minutes 4 servings

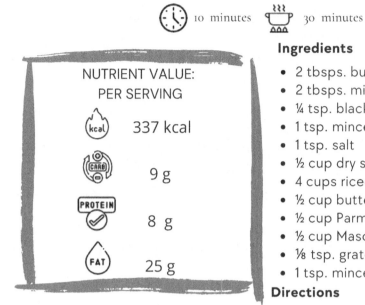

NUTRIENT VALUE:
PER SERVING

337 kcal

9 g

8 g

25 g

Ingredients

- 2 tbsps. butter
- 2 tbsps. minced sage
- ¼ tsp. black pepper, ground
- 1 tsp. minced rosemary
- 1 tsp. salt
- ½ cup dry sherry
- 4 cups riced cauliflower
- ½ cup butternut squash, cooked and mashed
- ½ cup Parmesan cheese, grated
- ½ cup Mascarpone cheese
- ⅛ tsp. grated nutmeg
- 1 tsp. minced garlic

Directions

- Melt your butter inside of a large frying pan turned to a medium level of heat.
- Add your rosemary, your sage, and garlic. Cook this for about 1 minute or until this mixture begins to become fragrant.
- Add in the cauliflower rice, pepper, salt, and mashed squash. Cook this for 3 minutes. You will know it is ready for the next step when cauliflower starts to soften up for you.
- Add in your sherry and cook this for an additional 6 minutes, or until the majority of the liquid is absorbed into the rice, or when the cauliflower is much softer.
- Stir in the Mascarpone cheese, Parmesan cheese, as well as nutmeg (grated).
- Cook all of this on a medium heat level, being sure to stir it occasionally, and do this until the cheese has melted and the risotto has gotten creamy. That will take around 20 minutes.
- Taste the risotto and add more pepper and salt to season if you wish.
- Remove your pan from the burner and garnish your risotto with more of the herbs as well as some grated parmesan.
- Serve and enjoy

RECIPES
SOUP
&
STEWS

1.CREAMY BROCCOLI AND CAULIFLOWER SOUP

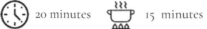 20 minutes   15 minutes   6 servings

NUTRIENT VALUE: PER SERVING

 264 kcal

 10 g

 7 g

 24 g

Ingredients

- 6 green onions
- ¼ tsp. ground white pepper
- (13½ oz./383g) 1 can unsweetened coconut milk
- 1 tsp gray sea salt
- ⅓ cup butter-infused olive oil
- 2 cups vegetable stock
- 1 (14 oz./397g) cauliflower florets
- 1 chopped green onion
- 2 celery sticks
- ¼ tsp. ground black pepper
- 1 head of broccoli florets

Directions

- Put a pan over medium flame.
- Now add in the coconut milk, vegetable stock, celery, salt, green onions, and cauliflower florets.
- Gently combine them, then cover and heat the soup till it boils.
- The soup needs another 15 minutes of simmering to soften the cauliflower florets.
- Broccoli should be blanched in a kettle of boiling water for one minute, while it is tender but still crisp, and then it should be drained on paper towels. On a dish, set aside.
- Transfer the prepared cauliflower soup to a blender.
- Olive oil, white and black pepper should be added. The soup should be well blended for a minute and a half.
- Blend once more for 30 seconds Now added the tender broccoli.
- Divide the cooked broccoli and cauliflower soup into 6 serving bowls.
- Garnish with chopped green onions and serve warm.

2.CHICKEN TURNIP SOUP

10 minutes   6 to 8 hours   5 servings

NUTRIENT VALUE: PER RECIPE

186 kcal

4 g

15 g

14 g

Ingredients

- 2 bay leaves
- 4 garlic cloves
- 4 cups water
- 3 thyme sprigs
- ¼ cup turnip
- ¼ cup onions
- Salt, to taste
- ¼ tsp. freshly ground black pepper
- 12 oz. (340g) bone-in chicken

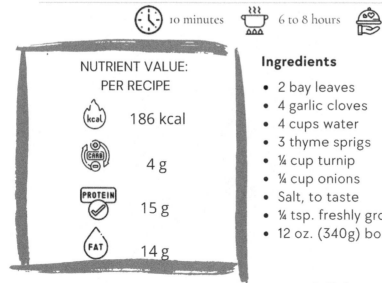

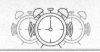

Directions:

- In a slow cooker, combine the chicken, turnip, onions, garlic, water, bay leaves, and thyme sprigs.
- After seasoning with salt along with pepper, thoroughly whisk the mixture.
- Cook the chicken completely on low for between six and eight hours with the cover on.
- When ready, remove the bay leaves and shred the chicken with a fork.
- Divide the soup among 5 bowls and serve.

3. GARLICKY CHICKEN SOUP

10 minutes   10 minutes   4 servings

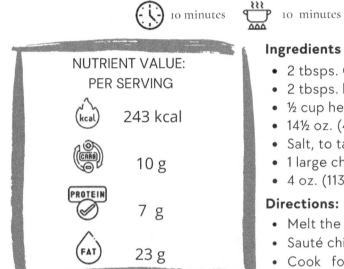

NUTRIENT VALUE:
PER SERVING

243 kcal

10 g

7 g

23 g

Ingredients

- 2 tbsps. Garlic Gusto Seasoning
- 2 tbsps. butter
- ½ cup heavy cream
- 14½ oz. (411 g) chicken broth
- Salt, to taste
- 1 large chicken breast
- 4 oz. (113 g) cream cheese

Directions:

- Melt the butter inside a pan over a moderate flame.
- Sauté chicken strips for 2 minutes.
- Cook for three minutes, stirring regularly, after adding cream cheese and salt.
- Now add in the chicken broth and heavy cream.
- After letting the soup boil for 4 minutes, season with salt.
- Let cool for 5 minutes and serve while warm.

4. CAULIFLOWER CURRY SOUP

15 minutes   26 minutes   4 servings

NUTRIENT VALUE:
PER SERVING

 342kcal

 7 g

 18 g

 29 g

Ingredients

- 2 tbsps. avocado oil
- 1 can unsweetened coconut milk
- 1 white onion
- 2 tsp. curry powder
- ¼ tsp. turmeric powder
- 4 garlic cloves
- 1 cup chicken broth
- 1 tsp. salt
- 1 cauliflower florets
- 1 cup water
- ½ serrano pepper
- Cilantro, for garnish
- 1-inch ginger
- ½ tsp. black pepper

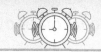

Directions:

- Sauté onions for three minutes in heated oil.
- Ginger, Serrano pepper, and garlic are added in the same pan, and they are sautéed for 2 minutes.
- Salt, black pepper, curry powder, and turmeric should be added. Following a moderate swirl, cook for 1 minute.
- After this add water and cauliflower in it and leave it to cook for ten minutes while covering the pan.
- The soup should be taken off the stove and let to cool to room temperature.
- Put this soup in a blender, and then puree it till it is smooth.
- Pour broth along with coconut milk into the soup after it has been returned to the pan. Cook for ten minutes.
- Divide the soup into 4 bowls and sprinkle the cilantro on top for garnish before serving.

5. BEEF TACO SOUP

 15 minutes 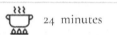 24 minutes 8 servings

NUTRIENT VALUE:
PER SERVING

 205 kcal

 8 g

 5 g

 13 g

Ingredients

- 1 tbsp. ground cumin
- 2 (14½ oz./411g) cans of beef broth
- 2 tsp. salt
- 2 (10 oz./284g) cans tomatoes and green chilies
- ½ cup heavy cream
- ½ cup onions
- 1 lb. (454 g) ground beef
- 2 garlic cloves
- 1 tsp. chili powder
- 1 (8 oz./227g) package of cream cheese

Directions:

- Put a pan on a medium-high flame.
- To the broth, now adds the garlic, onions, then ground beef. Sauté for 7 minutes, or till the meat is browned.
- Cook for two minutes then add cumin and chili powder.
- Cream cheese should be added and cooked for five minutes while being mashed into the meat with a spoon.
- Now add in tomatoes and green chilies, heavy cream, salt, and broth then cook for 10 minutes.
- Mix gently and serve warm.

6. CREAMY TOMATO SOUP

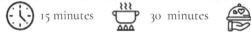 15 minutes 30 minutes 4 servings

Ingredients

- 1 cup heavy whipping cream
- 14 leaves of fresh basil
- 3 tomatoes, seeded and

- 4 cups tomato juice
- 2 tbsps. butter
- Salt and black pepper

- 2 cups water

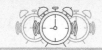
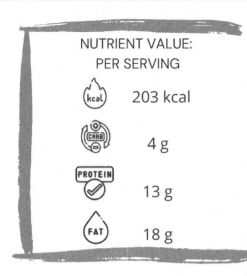

NUTRIENT VALUE:
PER SERVING

203 kcal

4 g

13 g

18 g

Directions:
- Take a cooking vessel that will work and set it on medium flame.
- After thirty minutes of simmering add water, tomato juice, then tomatoes.
- Now add in basil leaves after transferring the soup to a blender.
- Pulse the soup till it is smooth by using the pulse button.
- Put this tomato soup back in the pan and heat it to medium.
- Black pepper, salt, and heavy cream should all be added. Up till the butter melts, cook and blend.
- Serve warm and fresh.

7. CREAMY BROCCOLI AND LEEK SOUP

 5 minutes 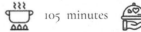 25 minutes 4 servings

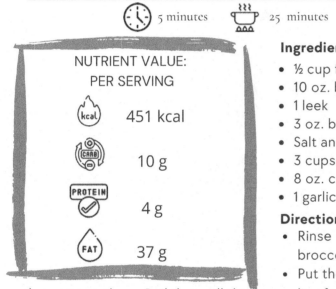

NUTRIENT VALUE:
PER SERVING

451 kcal

10 g

4 g

37 g

Ingredients
- ½ cup fresh basil
- 10 oz. broccoli
- 1 leek
- 3 oz. butter
- Salt and pepper
- 3 cups water
- 8 oz. cream cheese
- 1 garlic clove

Directions:
- Rinse the leek and chop both parts finely. Slice the broccoli thinly.
- Put the veggies inside a pan filled with water and then season them. Boil them till the broccoli softens.
- Now add in the florets and garlic, while lowering the heat.
- Now add in the cheese, butter, pepper, and basil. Blend till desired consistency: if too thick use water; if you want to make it thicker, use a little bit of heavy cream.

8. CHICKEN SOUP

25 minutes   105 minutes   4 servings

Ingredients
- 1 bay leaf
- 1 tsp. peppercorns
- 1 leek
- 1 chicken
- ½ cup white wine, dry
- 6 cups water
- Salt and pepper

- 1 medium carrot
- 1 yellow onion
- 2 garlic cloves
- 1 tbsp. thyme
-

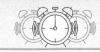
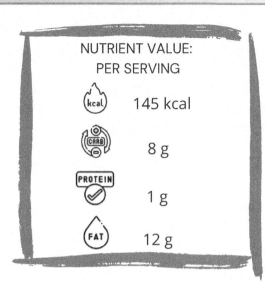

NUTRIENT VALUE: PER SERVING

kcal	145 kcal
CARB	8 g
PROTEIN	1 g
FAT	12 g

Directions:

- Peel and cut your veggies. Brown them in oil in a big pot.
- Split your chicken in half, down in the middle. Pour water and spices into the pot. Let it simmer for 1 hour.
- Take out the chicken save the meat, and toss away the bones.
- Put the meat back in the pot, and let it simmer on medium flame for 20-25 minutes again, while seasoning to your liking.

9. WILD MUSHROOM SOUP

🕐 10 minutes   🍲 30 minutes   🍽 4 servings

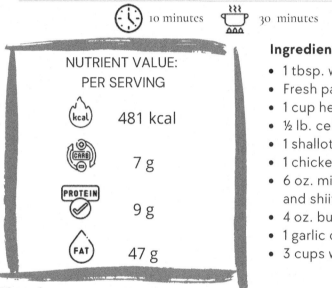

NUTRIENT VALUE: PER SERVING

kcal	481 kcal
CARB	7 g
PROTEIN	9 g
FAT	47 g

Ingredients

- 1 tbsp. white wine vinegar
- Fresh parsley
- 1 cup heavy whipping cream
- ½ lb. celery root
- 1 shallot
- 1 chicken bouillon cube
- 6 oz. mix portabella mushrooms, oyster mushrooms, and shiitake mushrooms
- 4 oz. butter
- 1 garlic clove
- 3 cups water

Directions:

- Clean, trim, and chop your mushrooms and celery. Do the same to your shallot and garlic.
- Sauté your chopped veggies in butter over medium flame in a pan.
- Now add in thyme, vinegar, chicken bouillon cube, and water then boil them. After some time let it simmer for fifteen minutes.
- Now add in the cream with an immersion blender till your desired consistency. Serve with parsley on top.

10. ROASTED BUTTERNUT SQUASH SOUP

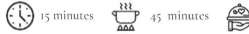 15 minutes   45 minutes   🍽 4 servings

Ingredients

- 25 oz. chicken broth
- 1 tbsp. fresh thyme
- 1 large butternut squash
- 3 tbsps. olive oil

- Salt and pepper
- 1 stalk celery
- 2 potatoes
- 1 large carrot

- 1 onion
- 1 tbsp. butter

 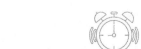

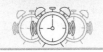

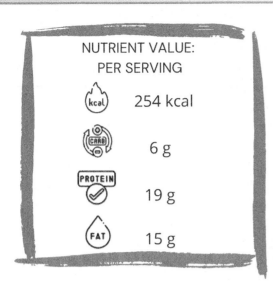

NUTRIENT VALUE:
PER SERVING

kcal 254 kcal

CARB 6 g

PROTEIN 19 g

FAT 15 g

Directions:

- Set the oven to 400 °F. Squash and potatoes should be tossed with 2 tablespoons of oil and seasoning on a baking sheet. For 20 to 25 minutes, roast.
- Melt the butter as well as the remaining oil inside a pan. Cook the onion, celery, as well as a carrot for five minutes. Also, season them.
- Now add in roasted potatoes and squash. The chicken broth should then be added. Use an immersion blender to simmer it for ten minutes to make the soup creamy.
- Garnish it with thyme.

11. ZUCCHINI CREAM SOUP

 5 minutes ♨ 20 minutes 🍲 4 servings

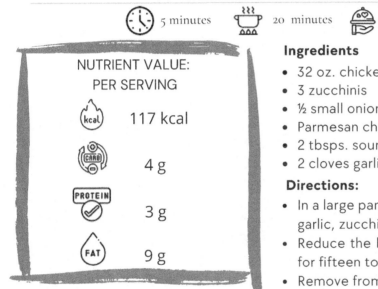

NUTRIENT VALUE:
PER SERVING

kcal 117 kcal

CARB 4 g

PROTEIN 3 g

FAT 9 g

Ingredients

- 32 oz. chicken broth
- 3 zucchinis
- ½ small onion
- Parmesan cheese
- 2 tbsps. sour cream
- 2 cloves garlic

Directions:

- In a large pan over medium flame, combine the broth, garlic, zucchini, then onion. Cook till boiling.
- Reduce the heat, cover, then let the mixture simmer for fifteen to twenty minutes.
- Remove from heat, Now add in the sour cream, then puree till smooth using a blender.
- Season to taste and top with your cheese.

12. CAULI SOUP

 5 minutes 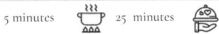 25 minutes 6 servings

Ingredients

- Grated parmesan
- 1 onion
- Salt and pepper

- 32 oz. vegetable broth
- 1 head cauliflower
- 2 garlic cloves

- ½ tbsp. olive oil
- green onion

Directions:

- Onion and garlic should now be added to the oil being heated over medium-low heat. Cook them for a further four to five minutes.
- Now add in the veggie broth and the cauliflower. Boil it, then leave it covered for fifteen to twenty minutes.

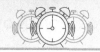

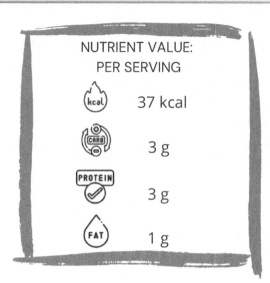

NUTRIENT VALUE:
PER SERVING

37 kcal

3 g

3 g

1 g

- Blend the entire pot's contents in a blender, then season it.
- Till smooth, blend. Now add in your cheese as well as green onion on the top.

13. THAI COCONUT SOUP

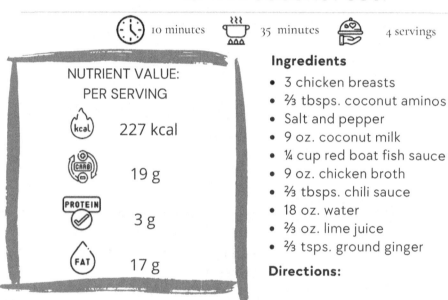

🕐 10 minutes   🍲 35 minutes   🍽 4 servings

NUTRIENT VALUE:
PER SERVING

227 kcal

19 g

3 g

17 g

Ingredients
- 3 chicken breasts
- ⅔ tbsps. coconut aminos
- Salt and pepper
- 9 oz. coconut milk
- ¼ cup red boat fish sauce
- 9 oz. chicken broth
- ⅔ tbsps. chili sauce
- 18 oz. water
- ⅔ oz. lime juice
- ⅔ tsps. ground ginger

Directions:

- Slice up the chicken breasts thinly. Make them bite-sized.
- In a stockpot, mix your coconut milk, water, fish sauce, chili sauce, lime juice, ginger, coconut aminos, and broth. Bring to a boil.
- Stir in chicken pieces. Lower the heat then cover the pot, while simmering it for half an hour.
- Remove basil leaves and season the soup.

RECIPES MEAT

1. MEATBALLS WITH KETO SAUCE

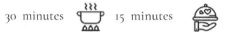

🕐 30 minutes   🍲 15 minutes   🍽 4 servings

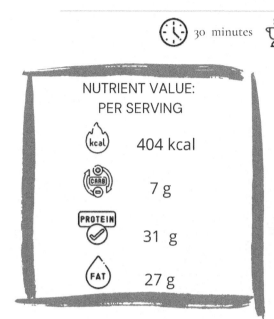

NUTRIENT VALUE:
PER SERVING

🔥 (kcal) 404 kcal

(CARB) 7 g

(PROTEIN) ✓ 31 g

(FAT) 27 g

Ingredients

- 1/2 cup (120 g) Parmesan cheese
- 2 tbsp. (30 g) heavy whipping cream
- 1 egg
- 1/2 cup (120 g) mozzarella cheese
- 1 clove garlic
- 1 pound (450 g) ground beef

Directions

- Set the temperature of the oven to 350°F.
- Combine egg, heavy whipping cream, Parmesan cheese, mozzarella cheese, and garlic in amixing basin.
- Lean ground beef should be added to the bowl after the other ingredients have been lightly but completely combined.
- Shape the mixture to form 1-1/2-inch meatballs, then arrange them on an oven rack in a 15x10x1-inch baking pan that has been oiled.
- The meatballs should be cooked appropriately and golden brown after twenty minutes in the oven.
- Prepare the sauce by mixing the prepared pesto, basil, garlic, oregano tomato sauce, and heavy whipping cream inside the pan while the meatballs are baking.
- The sauce should be brought to a boil after which it should be simmered till it thickens.
- Serve the cooked meatballs with the sauce drizzled for a delicious and creamy flavor.

2. SMOTHERED TURKEY

🕐 10 minutes   🍲 20 minutes   🍽 3 servings

NUTRIENT VALUE:
PER RECIPE

🔥 (kcal) 203 kcal

(CARB) 3 g

(PROTEIN) ✓ 27 g

(FAT) 9 g

Ingredients

- 2 slices provolone cheese
- 4 turkey breast halves (150 g each)
- 1 cup (200 g) fresh mushrooms
- 2 tsp (10 ml) olive oil
- A pinch of. (3 g) rotisserie turkey seasoning
- 1/4 cup (30 g) pecans
- 5 cups (700 g) fresh baby spinach
- 3 green onions

Directions:

- Get the broiler ready. Sliced mushrooms and green onions are cooked in olive oil - till they are soft.
- Fresh baby spinach, pecans, and other ingredients are stirred until the spinach wilts while the flavors are nicely blended.
- Keep the mushroom mix warm after turning off the stove.
- With rotisserie turkey seasoning, flavor the turkey breast halves to your liking.
- Cook the seasoned turkey in the broiler, 4 inches from the source. Cook for roughly four to five minutes on each side.
- After cooking, add half a piece of low-fat provolone cheese to each turkey breast.
- Place the turkey back under the grill or broiler to make the cheese gooey and wonderful.
- When ready to serve, dollop the tasty and nourishing mushroom mixture on the turkey breasts.

3. RUBBED TURKEY TS

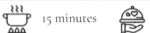 5 minutes   15 minutes   6 servings

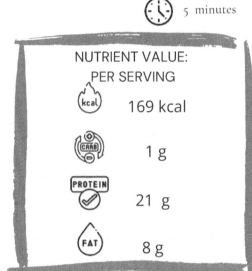

NUTRIENT VALUE:
PER SERVING

kcal   169 kcal

CARB   1 g

PROTEIN   21 g

FAT   8 g

Ingredients

- A pinch of. (3 g) sea salt
- 6 boneless, skinless turkeys (about 600 g)
- Pinch of (1 g) chili powder
- A pinch of. (3 g) garlic powder
- Pinch of (1 g) black pepper
- A pinch of. (3 g) onion powder
- Pinch of (1 g) paprika
- A pinch of. (3 g) turmeric powder
- A pinch of. (3 g) oregano

Directions:

- To produce the savory seasoning blend, sea salt, combine the chili powder, garlic powder, paprika, oregano, turmeric powder, onion powder, and black pepper in a bowl.
- To ensure that each piece of turkey gets the taste, evenly sprinkle the spice mixture across both sides of the turkey.
- Prepare the grill or the broiler too. To keep the grill rack from sticking, lightly oil it.
- The seasoned turkey may be broiled or grilled with the lid on aflame. Each side usually takes 6 to 8 minutes to cook the turkey until a thermometer placed into the thickest section registers 75°C (165°F).
- Once the turkey is cooked through, with a deliciously seasoned exterior, remove them from the grill or broiler and serve immediately. Enjoy the juicy and tender turkey is bursting with flavor from the well-balanced spice blend

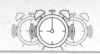
4. TS OF TURKEY WITH SHALLOTS AND SPINACH

 10 minutes   20 minutes   6 servings

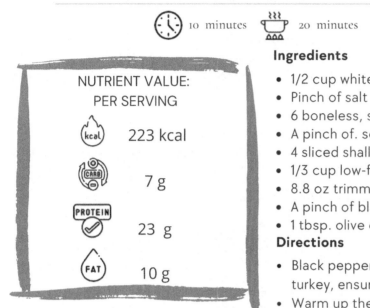

NUTRIENT VALUE:
PER SERVING

223 kcal

7 g

23 g

10 g

Ingredients

- 1/2 cup white wine (120 ml)
- Pinch of salt
- 6 boneless, skinless turkeys (about 1.3 lbs / 600 g)
- A pinch of. seasoned salt
- 4 sliced shallots
- 1/3 cup low-fat sour cream (75 g)
- 8.8 oz trimmed fresh spinach (250 g)
- A pinch of black pepper
- 1 tbsp. olive oil (15 ml)

Directions

- Black pepper and seasoned salt are used to season the turkey, ensuring to c both sides thoroughly.
- Warm up the olive oil in a nonstick pan.
- Place the seasoned turkey inside the pan then cook for six minutes. Remove the turkey from the pan and place it aside to keep it warm.
- Finely sliced shallots should be cooked and stirred in the same pan till they are soft and have a hint of caramelization.
- Add the white wine, then gently bring it to a boil. Simmer it till the liquid has been cut in half.
- Stirring the pan while cooking the fresh spinach
- Sprinkle in the salt, and give it a gentle stir.
- Stir in the low-fat sour cream, creating a creamy and delicious sauce for the turkey and spinach.
- Serve the cooked turkey a bed of creamy spinach, and enjoy this delightful and healthy meal.

5. POT ROAST WITH FLAVOR

10 minutes   7 minutes   15 servings

NUTRIENT VALUE:
PER SERVING

 142 kcal

 3 g

 15 g

 7 g

Ingredients

- 1 envelope of salad dressing mix (Italian)
- 1/2 cup water (120 ml)
- 2 boneless beef chuck roasts (each 2.2 lbs / 1 kg)
- 1 package brown gravy mix
- Optional: fresh parsley
- 1 package ranch salad dressing mix

Directions:

- Put the boneless beef chuck roasts in a 5-quart (5 L) slow cooker.
- Mix all dressings with brown gravy then add water and stir to combine to make a delicious sauce.
- On the beef roasts in the slow oven, pour the sauce.

- Simmer in the slow cooker for seven to eight hours on the low setting.
- Once cooked, the vegetables should be soft and infused with the savory flavors of the dressing mix and gravy.
- If desired, sprinkle the dish with fresh parsley to add a burst of color and fresh taste.

6. PAN GRAVY WITH TURKEY CUTLETS

🕐 10 minutes　🍲 10 minutes　🍽 4 servings

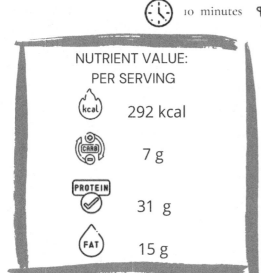

NUTRIENT VALUE:
PER SERVING

kcal 292 kcal

CARB 7 g

PROTEIN 31 g

FAT 15 g

Ingredients

- 2 tbsp. canola oil (30 ml)
- Pinch of pepper divided (1 g)
- 1 packet tenderloins of turkey breast (1.2 lbs / 550 g)
- 2 tbsp. melted butter (10 g)
- 1 pinch of turkey seasoning (3 g)
- 7 tbsp. all-purpose flour (100 g)
- 2 cups turkey stock (450 ml)
- Pinch of seasoned salt (1 g)

Directions:

- Slice the tenderloins of turkey breast into 1-inch slices crosswise. Flatten each piece with a meat mallet.
- Mix the seasoned salt, pepper, and turkey seasoning in a bowl.
- Over the slices of turkey, evenly distribute this spice mixture.
- Inside a pan, heat the canola oil on medium-high.
- Slices of seasoned turkey should be cooked in batches till no longer pink, taking approximately two minutes on each side. Take the cooked turkey out of the pan while keeping it warm.
- Butter should be melted over a low flame in the same pan. The mixture must be smooth and lump-free before adding the all-purpose flour. Pour the turkey stock gradually to make a delicious gravy.
- Cook and whisk the gravy for two minutes after boiling it.
- Add the remaining pepper to the gravy to season it.
- Serve the tenderloins of turkey breast with the delicious homemade gravy, adding a delightful flavor to the succulent turkey slices.

7. PROVOLONE TURKEY CHEESE

 5 minutes　 20 minutes　 4 servings

Ingredients

- 4 provolone cheese slices
- Pinch of pepper (1 g)
- Cooking spray scented with butter
- 4 turkey breast halves (4 pieces, 5 oz / 150 g each)
- 8 fresh basil leaves
- 4 slices prosciutto or deli ham, thinly sliced

Directions:

- Start by seasoning the turkey breast halves with a pinch of pepper, adding flavor to the dish.
- Use cooking spray that has a buttery fragrance and place the pan over the flame. It should take around four to five minutes on each side to cook the flavored turkey. Make sure the turkey is tender and thoroughly cooked.

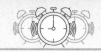
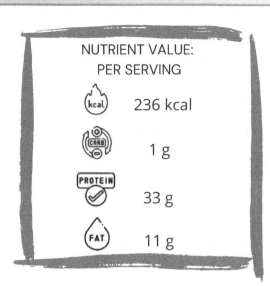

NUTRIENT VALUE:
PER SERVING

kcal   236 kcal

CARB   1 g

PROTEIN   33 g

FAT   11 g

- Transfer the cooked turkey breast halves to a baking sheet that hasn't been oiled. Top each piece of turkey with two fresh basil leaves, adding a delightful herbal aroma to the dish.
- Layer each turkey breast with thinly sliced prosciutto or deli ham, enhancing the flavor with savory goodness.
- Finally, Each turkey breast should have a piece of cheese. Broil the turkey six to eight inches from the flame for around two to three minutes until the cheese becomes seductively gooey and golden, producing a superb melted cheese finish.

8. ROASTED BEEF WITH GRAVY

 15 minutes   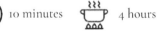 8 hours   10 servings

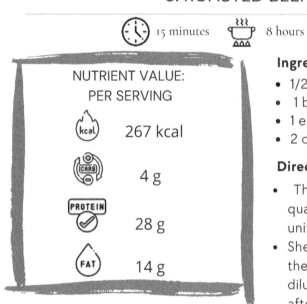

NUTRIENT VALUE:
PER SERVING

kcal   267 kcal

CARB   4 g

PROTEIN   28 g

FAT   14 g

Ingredients

- 1/2 cup (100 ml) sherry
- 1 boneless chuck roast beef (3.3 lbs / 1.5 Kg)
- 1 envelope of onion soup mix
- 2 cans (9.9 oz / 280 g each) cream of mushroom soup

Directions:

- The chuck roast should be split and placed in a 3-quart slow cooker. This guarantees tender results and uniform cooking.
- Sherry and the onion soup mix should be mixed with the cream of mushroom soup that has not been diluted. Pour the tasty mixture over the chuck roast after thoroughly mixing the ingredients.
- Set the slow cooker to low and allow the roast to cook for 8-10 hours. This slow-cooking process ensures that the beef becomes tender and succulent.
- After cooking, check the meat to ensure it is soft and fully cooked.
- Then serve the roast with the gravy and enjoy.

9. FOIL-WRAPPED POT ROAST

10 minutes   4 hours   8 servings

Ingredients

- 1 packet (dry) onion soup mix
- 3.3 lbs (1.5 kg) beef roast

- 10.5 oz (300 g) condensed cream of mushroom soup
- 0.7 fl oz (20 ml) water

Directions:

- Set the oven's temperature to 300 °F (150 °C).
- A 30-inch-long foil strip should be placed on the bottom of a 9 by 13-inch roasting pan.

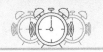
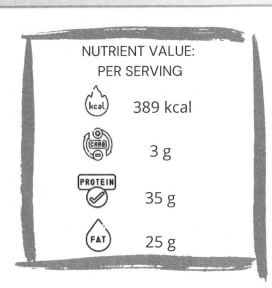

NUTRIENT VALUE:
PER SERVING

389 kcal

3 g

35 g

25 g

- Place the bottom round of the beef roast in the pan on the surface of the foil.
- Add onion soup mix, beef roast with cream of mushroom soup in the pan.
- Spray some water on the roast's surface.
- Fold the foil over the roast in half to form a sealed pouch and fasten the edges.
- Bake the roast within the foil package for four hours at 300°F (150°C).

10. BEEF TENDERLOIN WITH BLUE CHEESE

 30 minutes 1 hours 8 servings

NUTRIENT VALUE:
PER SERVING

669 kcal

5 g

35 g

54 g

Ingredients

- 4.2 fl oz (120 g) teriyaki sauce
- 3.3 lbs (1.5 kg) whole beef tenderloin
- 3.5 oz (100 g) sour cream
- 2 pinches of (5 g) Worcestershire sauce
- 1.9 cups (450 ml) red wine
- 4.2 oz (120 g) blue cheese
- 2 garlic cloves
- 3.5 oz (100 g) mayonnaise

Directions:

- Lay the entire beef tenderloin on a plate. Pour the red wine, garlic, and teriyaki sauce using a bowl. Pour the mix over the meat. Thirty minutes are enough for the heart to marinade in the refrigerator.
- The oven temperature is set at 450°F (230°C).
- The beef tenderloin should be placed on a broiler pan and then cooked in the oven for fifteen minutes. Once the desired degree of doneness is attained, lower the oven temperature to 375°F, then continue cooking for an additional forty minutes. Before slicing, let the steak 10 minutes to rest.
- Combine the blue cheese crumbles, mayonnaise, sour cream, and Worcestershire sauce in a low-heat pan. Stir the ingredients till it turns creamy and smooth.
- Slice the tenderloin then serve with blue cheese sauce drizzled on top.

11. BACON-WRAPS

 10 minutes 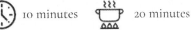 20 minutes 2 servings

Ingredients

- 5 bacon strips
- 10 stalks of fresh asparagus

- 1 pinch (1 g) black pepper
- Cooking spray

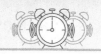
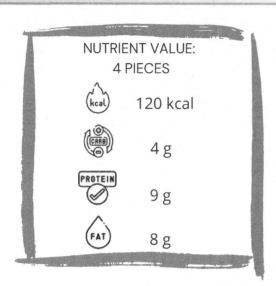

NUTRIENT VALUE:
4 PIECES

120 kcal

4 g

9 g

8 g

- Prepare the asparagus by trimming the tough ends. Put the asparagus on waxed paper and lightly spray them with cooking spray. Season with a pinch of black pepper and toss to coat evenly.
- Wrapping each half strip of bacon around a single asparagus spear, securing it in Put with a toothpick.
- Preheat your grill on flame.
- Grill the bacon-wrapped asparagus spears for about six minutes per side till the bacon turns crisp and the asparagus is tender.
- Take out the toothpicks from the asparagus spears before serving.

12. BAKED TURKEY

🕐 5 minutes   🍲 30 minutes   🍽 6 servings

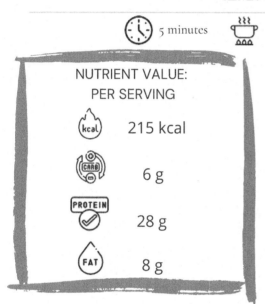

NUTRIENT VALUE:
PER SERVING

215 kcal

6 g

28 g

8 g

Ingredients
- 1 pinch (1 g) paprika
- 15 g butter
- 1 pinch (1 g) black pepper
- 250 g fresh mushrooms
- 120 g sherry or turkey broth
- 6 boneless, skinless turkey breast halves
- 1 pinch (2 g) salt
- 60 g part-skim mozzarella cheese,
- 3 green onions
- 1 garlic clove

Directions:
- Set your oven to 350°F (176°C). Cooking spray should be used to coat a 13x9-inch baking dish.
- Arrange the turkey breast halves inside the baking pan that has been prepared. Add a little paprika to the turkey.
- Bake the turkey for 15 minutes without the skin.
- Sliced mushrooms should be sautéed in butter in a nonstick skillet for five minutes until soft and lightly browned while the turkey bakes.
- Sherry or turkey broth, green onions, garlic, salt, and black pepper should all be combined in a bowl.
- After removing the turkey from the oven, cover it with the sherry or broth mix.
- Then put it inside the oven again and cook the turkey for ten more minutes.
- The part-skim mozzarella cheese should be sprinkled over the turkey before baking for three to five minutes until the cheese is melted.
- Serve the deliciously tender turkey with the flavorful mushroom sauce on top.

13. SLOW–COOKER TURKEY WITH HERBS

 5 minutes 4 minutes 4 servings

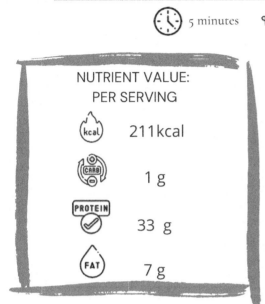

NUTRIENT VALUE:
PER SERVING

211 kcal

1 g

33 g

7 g

Ingredients

- 1 pinch of (2 g) thyme
- 1 pinch of (5 ml) olive oil
- 1 pinch of (2 g) black pepper
- Optional: ½ tsp. (3 ml) browning sauce
- 2 tbsp. (10 g) paprika
- 4 bone-in turkey breast halves
- ½ cup (120 ml) turkey broth
- 1 pinch of (2 g) garlic powder
- 1 pinch of (2 g) seasoned salt
- 1 pinch of (2 g) basil

Directions

- Seasoned salt, Olive oil, thyme, paprika, black pepper, basil, and garlic powder, with optional browning sauce, should all be combined in a bowl.
- With paper towels, rub the turkey dry. Turkey pieces should be uniformly coated with the prepared spice mixture by rubbing it in.
- Pour the turkey broth into a 5-quart slow cooker, filling it halfway.
- Put the seasoned turkey breast halves into the slow cooker, arranging them in a single layer.
- Cook the turkey in the slow cooker on the lowest setting possible for four to five hours until it is soft and cooked. Cover the slow cooker.
- Once the turkey is done, you can serve it as it is or pair it with your favorite side dishes for a delicious and satisfying meal.

14. MEAT TACOS

 10 minutes 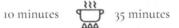 35 minutes 6 servings

NUTRIENT VALUE:
PER SERVING

 113 kcal

 2 g

 10 g

 7 g

Ingredients

- 1 tbsp. (20 g) salt
- 1 pinch of (3 g) cumin
- 1 pinch of (2 g) garlic powder
- 2 sliced onions
- 3.3 pounds (1.5 kg) of ground beef
- ½ tsp. (2 g) crushed red pepper flakes
- 2 cups (450 ml) water
- 3 tbsp. (20 g) chili powder

Directions:

- Cook the beef with thinly sliced onions over high heat inside a Dutch oven till the meat is no more pink. Excess fat in the pan should be drained.

- Add the salt, cumin, chili powder, garlic powder, and red pepper flakes to the meat mixture and the water. To ensure that the spices are spread equally, stir everything together.
- The mixture should be heated till it boils.
- Once the chili begins to boil, let it simmer for approximately fifteen minutes on low heat. Till the liquid becomes more concentrated and the aromas start to blend.
- Serve the mouthwatering homemade chili in bowls and, if you wish, sprinkle with cheese, sour cream, green onions, or jalapeño slices.

15. TENDERLOIN OF PEPPER-CRUSTED PORK

🕐 25 minutes   🍲 30 minutes   🤲 6 servings

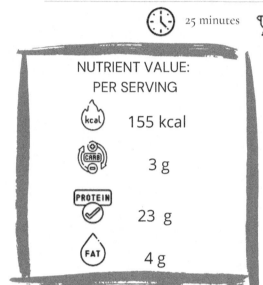

NUTRIENT VALUE:
PER SERVING

(kcal) 155 kcal

(CARB) 3 g

(PROTEIN) 23 g

(FAT) 4 g

Ingredients
- 2 pork tenderloins
- Salt: Pinch of (1 g)
- Dijon mustard: 3 tbsp. (45 g)
- Coarsely ground pepper: 1 pinch of (5 g)
- Fresh thyme: 1 tbsp. (8 g)
- Buttermilk: 1 pinch of (5 ml)
- Soft bread crumbs: 1 cup (100 g)

Directions:
- The oven temperature is set at 425°F (215°C).
- The savory mustard mixture is made by mixing the Dijon mustard, buttermilk thyme, roughly ground pepper, and salt in a basin.
- Make a double roast. Then, tie the tenderloins together using kitchen string at 1-1/2-inch spacing by placing them side by side with their thick ends touching.
- Using a 15x10x1-inch baking sheet, arrange the knotted tenderloins on a rack.
- Spread the tenderloins with the soft bread crumbs, carefully pressing them to cling to the mustard mix.
- A thermometer put into the thickest portion of the pork should read 150°F (65°C) after roasting the pork tenderloins in the oven for 30 to 40 minutes. To avoid browning, you can loosely tent the tenderloins with foil if necessary.
- Before slicing, let the cooked pork tenderloins rest for 5 minutes. Before cutting it, make sure to pull out the kitchen thread.

RECIPES
FISH

1.HALIBUT BLACKENED

🕐 5 minutes   🍲 20 minutes   🍽 4 servings

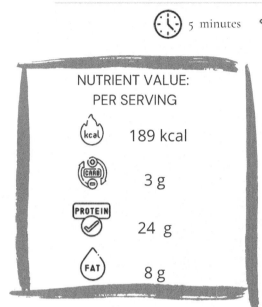

NUTRIENT VALUE:
PER SERVING

kcal 189 kcal

CARB 3 g

PROTEIN 24 g

FAT 8 g

Ingredients

- 0.7 ounces (20 g) Garlic powder
- 0.1 ounces (3 g) Salt
- 0.1 ounces (3 g) Onion powder
- 0.4 ounces (10 g) Dried oregano
- 0.1 ounces (3 g) Dried thyme
- 0.4 ounces (10 g) Cayenne pepper
- 0.1 ounces (3 g) Pepper
- 0.9 ounces (25 g) Paprika
- 3.9 ounces (110 g) each Halibut fillet (4 fillets, about)
- 1.1 ounces (30 g) Melted butter

Directions

- Paprika, garlic powder, dried thyme, dried oregano, salt, and cayenne pepper should all be combined in a bowl.
- The halibut fillets should be equally covered on both sides with the spice mixture.
- The grill pan should be heated to medium-high.
- Please ensure the halibut fillets are well-coated with the melted butter by drizzling them over them.
- Put the halibut fillets onto the grill pan after seasoning.
- The fillets on each side should be cooked through and flaky for around 3 to 4 minutes.
- Halibut fillets are taken off the grill and placed on serving trays.
- The grilled halibut fillets with your preferred side dishes should be given as soon as possible.

2. RED SNAPPER WITH CRUMB COATING

🕐 10 minutes   🍲 20 minutes   🍽 4 servings

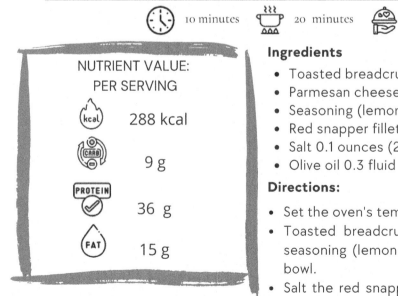

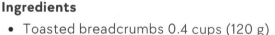

NUTRIENT VALUE:
PER SERVING

kcal 288 kcal

CARB 9 g

PROTEIN 36 g

FAT 15 g

Ingredients

- Toasted breadcrumbs 0.4 cups (120 g)
- Parmesan cheese, grated 1 ounce (30 g)
- Seasoning (lemon pepper) 0.1 ounces (3 g)
- Red snapper fillets 4 fillets
- Salt 0.1 ounces (2 g)
- Olive oil 0.3 fluid ounces (10 ml)

Directions:

- Set the oven's temperature to 392°F (200°C).
- Toasted breadcrumbs, grated Parmesan cheese, and seasoning (lemon pepper) should all be combined in a bowl.
- Salt the red snapper fillets on both sides after patting them dry with a paper towel.

- Olive oil should be gently brushed on each fillet.
- Each fillet's top side should be evenly coated with the bread crumb mix after being pressed onto it.
- Put the coated fillets on a parchment paper–lined baking sheet.
- For approximately ten to twelve minutes, until the fish is opaque and flakes readily with a fork, bake inside the oven.
- Red snapper fillets that have been roasted should be served right away.

3. FILLETS OF HERB-ROASTED SALMON

 5 minutes   25 minutes   4 servings

NUTRIENT VALUE:
PER SERVING

 301 kcal

 1 g

 29 g

 19 g

Ingredients

- 1 teaspoon (5 ml) Olive oil
- 4 fillets (130 g each) Fillets of salmon
- 4 cloves Minced garlic cloves
- 0.5 tablespoons (15 g) Minced fresh rosemary OR Crushed dried rosemary: 0.5 tablespoons (15 g)
- 0.03 ounces (1 g) Salt
- 2 teaspoons (10 g) OR Dried thyme: 1 teaspoon (3 g) Fresh minced thyme
- 0.07 ounces (2 g) Black pepper

Directions:

- Set the oven's temperature to 392 F - (200 C).
- To make a marinade, combine the minced garlic, fresh or dried rosemary, olive oil, fresh or dried thyme, salt, and black pepper in a small bowl.
- The salmon fillets should be placed into a baking dish.
- Each salmon fillet should have the marinade uniformly applied.
- For the salmon to fully absorb the spices, marinade it for fifteen to twenty minutes.
- For about twelve to fifteen minutes, till the salmon flakes effortlessly with a fork or is cooked to your preferred level of doneness, bake the salmon inside the preheated oven.
- Once done, please take the salmon out of the oven, then serve with more fresh herbs as a garnish, if you'd like.

4. QUICK SALMON PATTIES

 10 minutes   15 minutes   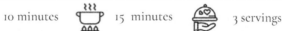 3 servings

Ingredients

- 0.35 cups (100 g) Finely chopped onion
- 1 large Beaten egg
- 5 pieces Crushed saltines
- 0.08 fluid ounces (2 ml) Worcestershire sauce

- 0.03 ounces (1 g) Salt
- 0.03 ounces (1 g) Black pepper
- 1 can (400 g), bones and skin removed Drained salmon
- 1.06 ounces (30 g) Melted butter

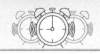

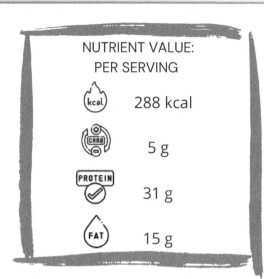

**NUTRIENT VALUE:
PER SERVING**

288 kcal

5 g

31 g

15 g

Directions:
- Set the oven's temperature to 180 C (356 F).
- The finely diced onion, beaten egg, saltines, Worcestershire sauce, salt, and black pepper should all be combined in a mixing bowl. Mix thoroughly.
- Salmon that has been drained should be added to the bowl and then carefully mixed with the remaining ingredients.
- Create the proper size patties out of the ingredients.
- Melted butter should be heated over medium heat in a pan.
- The salmon patties should be carefully placed in the pan and cooked on both sides for three to four minutes until they are light brown and thoroughly done.
- Or, if you'd instead bake them, spread the salmon patties out on a baking sheet covered with parchment paper. Cook and properly brown them in the oven for fifteen to twenty minutes, turning them halfway through.
- When the salmon patties have finished cooking, take them from the pan or oven and give them time to rest before serving.
- With your preferred side dishes, such as a crisp salad or steamed vegetables, serve the salmon patties.

5. FILLETS OF SEASONED TILAPIA

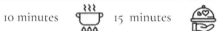 10 minutes 15 minutes 2 servings

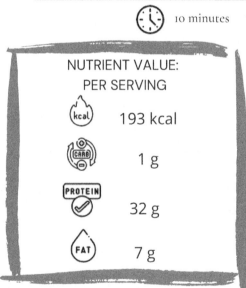

**NUTRIENT VALUE:
PER SERVING**

193 kcal

1 g

32 g

7 g

Ingredients
- 2 fillets (150 g each) Tilapia fillets
- 0.53 ounces (15 g) Melted butter
- 0.18 ounces (5 g) Montreal steak seasoning
- 0.07 ounces (2 g) Flakes dried parsley
- 0.03 ounces (1 g) Paprika
- 0.03 ounces (1 g) Dried thyme
- 0.03 ounces (1 g) Onion powder
- 0.03 ounces (1 g) Pepper
- 0.03 ounces (1 g) Salt
- a pinch Garlic powder

Directions:
- Set the oven's temperature to 200 C (392 F).
- Put the tilapia fillets over an oven tray with aluminum foil or parchment paper.
- Melted butter, dried parsley, paprika, dried thyme, onion powder, pepper, and salt should all be combined in a small bowl with a dash of garlic powder.
- Tilapia fillets should be uniformly coated with the seasoned butter mixture on both sides.
- When the tilapia is cooked thoroughly and flakes easily with a fork, put the baking sheet in the oven that has been preheated and bake for twelve to fifteen minutes.
- Once done, take the tilapia fillets out of the oven and give them a few seconds to rest.
- Rice, steamed veggies, or any other side dish you choose should be served with tilapia fillets.
- Then serve and enjoy.

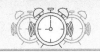
6. KABOBS OF GINGER–TUNA

 25 minutes   5 minutes   8 servings

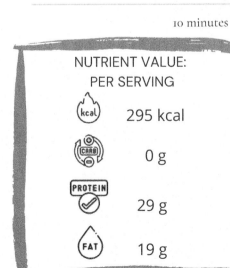

NUTRIENT VALUE:
PER SERVING

100 kcal

1 g

8 g

7 g

Ingredients

- 16 cubes tuna steaks (450 g)
- 0.5 fluid ounces soy sauce (15 ml)
- 1 fluid ounce rice vinegar (30 ml)
- 0.53 ounces toasted sesame seeds (15 g)
- 1 fluid ounce canola oil (30 ml)
- 0.1 ounces pepper (3 g)
- 16 slices pickled ginger
- 1 bunch watercress (optional)
- 4.23 ounces mayonnaise with wasabi (120 g)

Directions

- The tuna steaks should be cut into 16 pieces and kept aside.
- To make a marinade, mix 0.5 fluid ounces of soy sauce and 1 fluid ounce of rice vinegar in a basin.
- Add 0.1 ounces of pepper, 1 fluid ounce of canola oil, and 0.53 ounces of toasted sesame seeds to the marinade. Mix thoroughly.
- Tuna cubes should marinate for 15 to 20 minutes after being added to the marinade.
- Place slices of pickled ginger on a serving plate. Please prepare and add watercress and ginger if you'd like.
- The tuna cubes should be removed from the marinade and put on the dish.
- Pour some leftover marinade over the tuna cubes to give them more flavor.
- For richness and a touch of fire, serve with an additional layer of wasabi-infused mayonnaise.
- Garnish the tuna cubes with the watercress (if using) and slices of pickled ginger.
- Savor this delicious dish as an appetizer, a light main course, or a component of a sushi-themed meal.

7. SALMON OVEN–ROASTED

10 minutes   10 minutes   4 servings

NUTRIENT VALUE:
PER SERVING

295 kcal

0 g

29 g

19 g

Ingredients

- 1 center-cut salmon fillet (220 g)
- 0.17 fluid ounces of olive oil (5 ml)
- 0.07 ounces salt (2 g)
- 0.07 ounces pepper (2 g)

Directions:

- Set your oven's temperature to the correct level (typically around 200°C).
- The center-cut salmon fillet (220 g) should be put on a baking sheet or in a dish that can go in the oven.
- Over the salmon fillet, drizzle 0.17 fluid ounces (5 ml) of olive oil.

- Spread a thin layer of salt (0.07 ounces; 2 g) all over the fillet.
- With a uniform distribution, sprinkle 0.07 ounces (2 g) of pepper over the fillet.
- To help the spices stick to the fish, gently pat them on.
- Put a baking tray containing the salmon fillet in the already-heated oven.
- Depending on the thickness of the salmon and the degree of doneness you choose, bake it for the recommended time. For 2.5 cm of thickness, salmon is usually cooked for fifteen to twenty minutes.
- To avoid overcooking the fish, please keep an eye on it. With a fork, it ought should flake off opaquely.
- Take the salmon out of the oven after it is fully cooked.
- You can move the salmon fillet onto a serving plate with caution.
- If you would like, please pair it with fresh herbs, lemon slices, and your preferred sauce.
- Serve your tasty, flawlessly cooked salmon as the centerpiece of your meal with your preferred sides.

8. CITRUS SALMON

20 minutes  15 minutes 6 servings

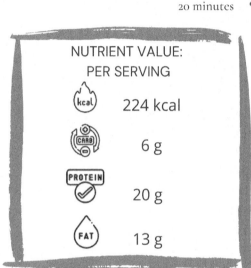

NUTRIENT VALUE:
PER SERVING

kcal   224 kcal

CARB   6 g

PROTEIN   20 g

FAT   13 g

Ingredients

- 6 orange wedges
- 6 lime wedges
- 6 fillets of salmon (110 g each)
- 1 pound fresh asparagus, trimmed and cut in half (450 g)
- Cooking spray scented with olive oil
- 0.07 ounces of salt (2 g)
- 0.035 ounces of pepper (1 g)
- 1 ounce fresh parsley, minced (30 g)
- 1.5 fluid ounces lemon juice (45 ml)

Directions:

- Set the oven to 200 °C (or 390 °F).
- On a baking sheet, arrange the orange and lime wedges to provide a bed for the salmon and asparagus.
- Over the citrus wedges, arrange the salmon fillets (110 g each).
- Place the salmon fillets in a circle around the asparagus half (1 pound or 450 g) on the baking tray.
- Spray some cooking spray with an olive oil aroma and lightly coat the fish and asparagus.
- Over the salmon and asparagus, equally distribute 0.07 ounces (2 g) of salt and 0.035 ounces (1 g) of pepper.
- The salmon should flake easily with a fork while the asparagus should be tender after roasting in the oven that has been preheated for twelve to fifteen minutes.
- Make the sauce while the fish and asparagus are roasting. 1 ounce (30 g) of finely chopped fresh parsley and 1.5 fluid ounces (45 ml) of lemon juice should be combined in a small basin.
- Take the salmon and the asparagus out of the oven after cooking.
- Serve the salmon fillets with asparagus on separate plates.
- Over the salmon, along with asparagus, drizzle the lemon-parsley sauce.
- Enjoy the savory fish, crisp asparagus, and tangy citrus flavors immediately by serving.

9. COD POACHED IN TOMATO BROTH

 5 minutes   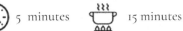 15 minutes   2 servings

NUTRIENT VALUE:
PER SERVING

 167 kcal

 1 g

 18 g

 10 g

Ingredients

- 450 grams fillet of wild-caught fish, cut into 3-inch squares
- 250 grams of organic whole peeled tomatoes
- 600 milliliters of pastured chicken broth
- Saffron, just a pinch (about 15 threads)
- Two bay leaves
- 45 milliliters avocado oil
- To taste, sea salt

Directions

- 45 milliliters of avocado oil should be warmed in a big saucepan over medium heat.
- 250 grams of whole, peeled organic tomatoes should be added to the saucepan. As they cook, use a spoon to break them apart.
- 600 milliliters of pastured chicken broth should be added, and the mixture should boil gently.
- 15 strands of saffron should be added to the saucepan as a pinch. This flavorful spice will give the stew a lovely golden hue and a delicate flavor.
- Add the two bay leaves for further flavor depth.
- Squares of wild-caught fish fillet (450 grams) should be carefully added to the boiling soup. Cook them for just a few minutes till they are opaque and well-cooked.
- Taste the stew while it simmers and add sea salt if desired. Remember that the bay leaves and saffron will also add to the overall taste profile.
- The stew is suitable to be consumed once the fish has finished cooking and the flavors have combined.
- Making sure that each dish has an equal amount of fish, tomatoes, and flavorful broth, dish the fish stew onto serving bowls.
- Serve the stew with complementary dishes or crusty bread that soaks up the flavorful liquid.

10. CHILI COD

 10 minutes   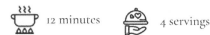 12 minutes   4 servings

Ingredients

- 4 cod fillets, boneless
- 2 tablespoons avocado oil
- A pinch of salt and black pepper
- 1 teaspoon chili powder
- 1 tablespoon cilantro, chopped
- 3 garlic cloves, minced
- ½ teaspoon chili pepper, crushed

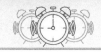

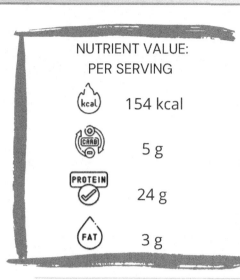

NUTRIENT VALUE:
PER SERVING

154 kcal

5 g

24 g

3 g

Directions:
- Heat up a pan with the oil over medium-high heat, add the garlic, chili pepper, and chili powder, stir and cook for 2 minutes.
- Add the fish and the other ingredients, cook for 5 minutes on each side, divide between plates, and serve.

11. PARSLEY TUNA BOWLS

 10 minutes 15 minutes 4 servings

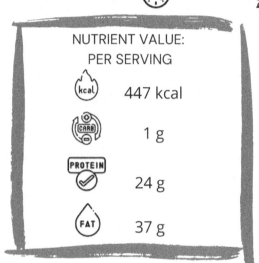

NUTRIENT VALUE:
PER SERVING

447 kcal

1 g

24 g

37 g

Ingredients
- 1 pound tuna fillets, boneless, skinless, and cubed
- 1 tablespoon olive oil
- 1 tablespoon parsley, chopped
- 2 scallions, chopped
- 1 tablespoon lime juice
- 1 teaspoon garlic powder
- A pinch of salt and black pepper

Directions:
- Heat the oil in a pan over medium-high heat, add the scallions, and sauté for 2 minutes.
- Add the fish and the other ingredients, toss gently, cook for 12 more minutes, divide into bowls, and serve.

RECIPES
SALADS

1. SALAD WITH CRISPY SPINACH

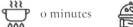 10 minutes — 0 minutes — 2 servings

Ingredients

- Shredded carrot, weighing around 4.23 ounces (120 grams)
- A portion of spinach, about 15.87 ounces (450 grams)
- Pumpkin seeds, approximately 0.35 ounces (10 grams)
- About 2 teaspoons (10 milliliters) of balsamic vinegar
- One small apple
- Two teaspoons (10 milliliters) of olive oil
- Diced cucumber, about 4.23 ounces (120 grams)
- Chopped plum tomato, included

Directions

- Wash and thoroughly dry the spinach.
- Chop the plum tomato (1) into bite-sized pieces then put it in a bowl.

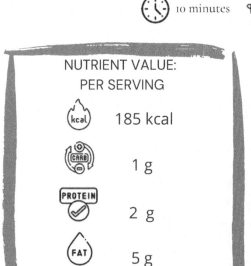

NUTRIENT VALUE:
PER SERVING

185 kcal

1 g

2 g

5 g

- Peel and dice a tiny apple (1), and incorporate it into the bowl.
- Slice the cucumber and add it to the mix for a refreshing crunch.
- Add the shredded carrot to enhance color and texture.
- Sprinkle the pumpkin seeds over the salad for added nuttiness and crunch.
- Drizzle the olive oil evenly over the salad.
- Follow with the balsamic vinegar for a tangy and rich flavor.
- Gently toss the ingredients to ensure an even distribution of flavors and textures.
- Serve immediately as a delightful and nutritious salad.

2. SALAD WITH A MINTY DRESSING FROM GREECE

 20 minutes 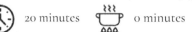 0 minutes 4 servings

Ingredients

- One small cucumber, diced, weighing approximately 0.22 pounds
- Chopped red pepper, amounting to about 0.22 pounds
- Chopped green pepper, also around 0.22 pounds.
- Sliced plum tomatoes totaling about 0.66 pounds
- Finely sliced green onions, a handful
- Crumbled feta cheese, roughly 3.53 ounces (about 100 grams)
- Two cloves of garlic
- About 3 tablespoons (approximately 45 milliliters) of olive oil

- Freshly squeezed lemon juice from 1 to 2 lemons
- Chopped mint, approximately 1.59 ounces (about 45 grams)
- Season with salt and pepper according to your taste

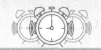
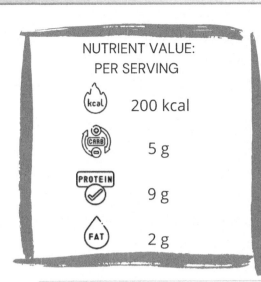

NUTRIENT VALUE:
PER SERVING

200 kcal

5 g

9 g

2 g

Directions:

- Combine diced cucumber, chopped red pepper, chopped green pepper, sliced plum tomatoes, and sliced green onions inside a bowl.
- Add crumbled feta and chopped mint to the bowl.
- Mix minced garlic cloves, olive oil, and lemon juice in a separate bowl. Adjust lemon juice quantity to taste.
- Over the salad, drizzle the dressing, and toss just enough to mix.
- To your liking, season using pepper as well as salt.
- Dispense and savor!

3. SALAD WITH ARUGULA

 10 minutes 0 minutes 4 servings

NUTRIENT VALUE:
PER SERVING

150 kcal

4 g

7 g

12 g

Ingredients

- A measurement of approximately 0.34 fluid ounces (10 milliliters) of balsamic vinegar
- Fresh arugula, weighing around 8.8 ounces (250 grams)
- Season with salt and pepper according to your preference
- Fresh strawberries total about 8.8 ounces (250 grams)
- Roughly 0.35 ounces (10 grams) of chopped pecans
- Two teaspoons (around 10 milliliters) of olive oil
- Finely sliced red onion, about 1 to 2 portions

Directions:

- Mix 250 g fresh arugula, sliced red onion, and fresh strawberries.
- Sprinkle with 10 g chopped pecans.
- Drizzle with 10 ml olive oil and 10 ml balsamic vinegar.
- Sprinkle salt n pepper then serve.

4. CHICKPEA BOOSTER BOWL

 10 minutes 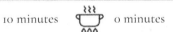 0 minutes 2 servings

Ingredients

- Roughly 1.76 ounces (50 grams) of diced cucumber
- About 0.53 ounces (15 grams) of plum tomato, thinly sliced
- Approximately 0.71 ounces (20 grams) of red onion
- Shredded carrot, amounting to around 1.76 ounces (50 grams)

- About 0.53 ounces (15 grams) of parsley
- Cleaned chickpeas weigh about 1.76 ounces (50 grams)
- A tablespoon (approximately 15 milliliters) of lemon juice
- Add salt and pepper to taste

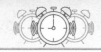

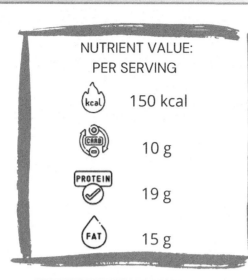

NUTRIENT VALUE:
PER SERVING

150 kcal

10 g

19 g

15 g

Directions:
- Mix chickpeas, shredded carrot, sliced plum tomato, chopped cucumber, red onion, and parsley.
- Drizzle with lemon juice.
- Sprinkle salt n pepper then serve.

5. HEART OF ROMAINE GRILLED

 10 minutes   10 minutes   4 servings

NUTRIENT VALUE:
PER SERVING

100 kcal

6 g

14 g

7 g

Ingredients
- A teaspoon of olive oil, measuring about 5 milliliters
- One romaine heart sliced lengthwise
- Half a fluid ounce of balsamic vinegar is roughly 15 milliliters
- Two tablespoons of lemon juice, equivalent to about 30 milliliters
- You can season with salt and pepper according to taste
- Approximately 1.76 ounces (50 grams) of cherry tomatoes
- Around 0.53 ounces (15 grams) of Parmesan cheese

Directions:
- On a platter, arrange the sliced romaine heart.
- Sprinkle the romaine with 2 tbsp of lemon juice
- Cherry tomatoes, 1.76 oz (50 g), should be sprinkled on top
- Add 15 g or 0.53 oz of Parmesan cheese
- Pour 15 ml (0.5 fl oz) of balsamic vinegar over the dish
- Serve after adding salt and pepper
- Add 0.17 fl oz (5 ml) of olive oil to finish

6. TUNA SALAD

 10 minutes   0 minutes   1 servings

Ingredients
- A measure of 2 tablespoons (approximately 30 milliliters) of olive oil
- A quantity of 2.8 ounces (around 80 grams) of tuna
- An amount of 7.05 ounces (200 grams) of assorted mixed greens
- Pinches of salt and pepper to season.
- About 1 tablespoon (approximately 15 milliliters) of lemon juice
- Around 1.06 ounces (30 grams) of cherry tomatoes
- Roughly 0.7 ounces (20 grams) of thinly sliced radish
- One green onion, finely sliced

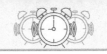

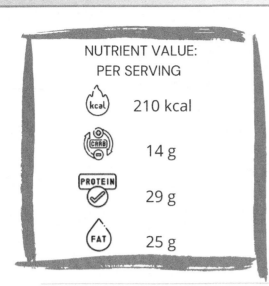

NUTRIENT VALUE:
PER SERVING

210 kcal

14 g

29 g

25 g

Directions:
- Tuna, mixed greens, cherry tomatoes, radish, and green onion should all be combined.
- Olive oil and lemon juice should be drizzled on.
- Serve after adding salt and pepper.

7. SALAD WITH CHICKEN AND ASPARAGUS

 3 minutes   4 minutes   2 servings

NUTRIENT VALUE:
PER SERVING

220 kcal

10 g

22 g

15 g

Ingredients
- A measure of approximately 0.34 fluid ounces (10 milliliters) of olive oil.
- Diced cooked chicken, weighing about 1.8 ounces (50 grams).
- Halved cherry tomatoes totaling around 1.8 ounces (50 grams).
- Asparagus spears, about 3.5 ounces (100 grams).
- Season with salt and pepper to taste.
- Crumbled feta cheese, roughly 0.35 ounces (10 grams).
- Half a fluid ounce (approximately 15 milliliters) of lemon juice.

Directions:
- Cherry tomatoes, feta cheese, asparagus, and chopped chicken should all be combined.
- Olive oil and lemon juice should be drizzled on.
- Serve after adding salt and pepper.

8. SALAD OF WATERMELON AND ARUGULA

 5 minutes   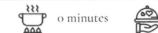 0 minutes   2 servings

Ingredients

- Diced watermelon, measuring approximately 3.5 ounces (100 grams)
- Arugula, weighing around 1.8 ounces (50 grams)
- Chopped red onion, roughly 0.7 ounces (20 grams)

- Crumbled feta cheese, about 0.7 ounces (20 grams)
- Half a fluid ounce (around 15 milliliters) of balsamic vinegar

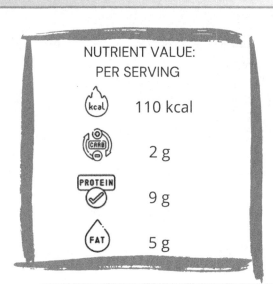

NUTRIENT VALUE:
PER SERVING

110 kcal

2 g

9 g

5 g

Directions:
- Toss diced watermelon, arugula, chopped red onion, and crumbled feta in a bowl.
- Drizzle with balsamic vinegar and mix gently.

9. TARRAGON SALAD

 5 minutes   5 minutes   4 servings

Ingredients

- Shredded light water-packed tuna, drained and weighing approximately 6.2 ounces (175 grams).
- Chopped celery, about 8.8 ounces (250 grams).
- Finely sliced sweet onion, around 2.6 ounces (75 grams).
- Low-fat mayonnaise, totaling about 3.5 ounces (100 grams).

- Minced fresh parsley, approximately 1 ounce (30 grams).
- About 0.17 fluid ounces (5 milliliters) of lemon juice.
- Chopped fresh tarragon, or about 0.18 ounces (5 grams) of dried tarragon.
- Dijon mustard, roughly 0.07 ounces (2 grams).
- Ground white pepper, around 0.03 ounces (1 gram).
- Optionally, serve with lettuce leaves.

Directions:
- The tuna, celery, and thinly sliced sweet onion should all be combined in a mixing dish after being drained and shredded.
- Mix the low-fat mayonnaise, fresh parsley that has been minced, lemon juice, tarragon that has been chopped, Dijon mustard, and white pepper in a separate bowl.
- Mix the tuna mixture with the dressing by pouring it over the top and gently tossing.
- If preferred, serve the tuna salad atop lettuce leaves as a light and tasty entrée.

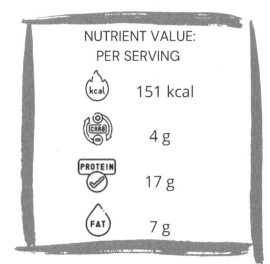

NUTRIENT VALUE:
PER SERVING

151 kcal

4 g

17 g

7 g

RECIPES
DESSERT

1. BAKED APPLES

 5 minutes 20 minutes 4 servings

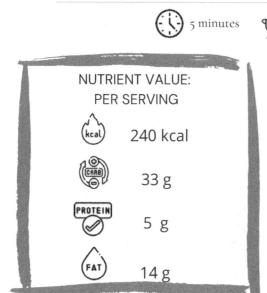

NUTRIENT VALUE:
PER SERVING

kcal — 240 kcal

CARB — 33 g

PROTEIN — 5 g

FAT — 14 g

Ingredients

- 4 apples, cored
- ¼ cup coconut oil, softened
- 4 tsp. ground cinnamon
- ⅛ tsp. ground ginger
- ⅛ tsp. ground nutmeg

Directions

- Preheat the oven to 350°F.
- Fill each apple with 1 tbsp. of coconut oil.
- Sprinkle with spices evenly.
- Apples should be arranged on a baking pan.
- For twelve to eighteen minutes, bake.

2. PUMPKIN ICE CREAM

 15 minutes  0 minutes 6 servings

NUTRIENT VALUE:
PER SERVING

kcal — 293 kcal

CARB — 25 g

PROTEIN — 2 g

FAT — 23 g

Ingredients

- 1½ tsp. pumpkin pie spice
- ½ tsp. ground cinnamon
- 15 oz. homemade pumpkin puree
- ½ cup dates
- A pinch of salt
- 2 (14-oz) cans of unsweetened coconut milk
- ½ tsp. organic vanilla extract

Directions:

- All the ingredients should be combined in a high-powered blender and blended until smooth.
- Frozen for around 1-2 hours after being transferred into an airtight container.
- Place the mixture in an ice cream machine at this point, and proceed by following the manufacturer's instructions.
- Before serving, put the ice cream back in the airtight container while freezing for a further hour or two.

3. AVOCADO PUDDING

 15 minutes 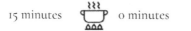 0 minutes 4 servings

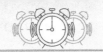
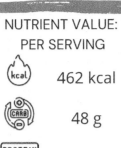

NUTRIENT VALUE:
PER SERVING

 462 kcal

 48 g

PROTEIN 3 g

FAT 20 g

Ingredients

- 1 tsp. fresh lime zest
- ⅓ cup agave nectar
- 1 tsp. fresh lemon zest
- 2 cups bananas
- ½ cup fresh lemon juice
- 2 ripe avocados
- ½ cup fresh lime juice

Directions:

- All the ingredients should be combined in a blender and pulsed until smooth.
- Before serving, place the mousse in flutes and place them in the refrigerator to cool for approximately three hours.

4. CHOCOLATE MOUSSE

 10 minutes 0 minutes 4 servings

NUTRIENT VALUE:
PER SERVING

 357 kcal

 52 g

PROTEIN 14 g

FAT 13 g

Ingredients

- 4 Medjool dates
- ½ cup unsweetened almond milk
- 4 tbsps. fresh blueberries
- 1 cup cooked black beans
- 1 tsp. organic vanilla extract
- ½ cup pecans
- 2 tbsps. non-alkalized cocoa powder

Directions:

- All the ingredients should be combined in a food processor and pulsed till they are smooth and creamy.
- Transfer the mixture to serving bowls and refrigerate to chill before serving.
- Garnish with blueberries and serve.

5. APPLE CRISP

 15 minutes 20 minutes 8 servings

Ingredients

For Filling:

- 2 large apples, peeled, cored, and chopped
- 2 tbsps. water
- 2 tbsps. fresh apple juice
- ¼ tsp. ground cinnamon

For Topping:

- ½ cup quick rolled oats
- ¼ cup unsweetened coconut flakes
- 2 tbsps. pecans
- ½ tsp. ground cinnamon
- ¼ cup water

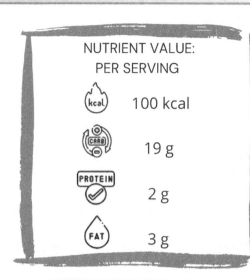

NUTRIENT VALUE:
PER SERVING

100 kcal

19 g

2 g

3 g

Directions:

- Turn the oven on to 300°F. Grease a baking pan very lightly.
- In a dish, combine all the filling ingredients and stir just until combined. Leave this alone.
- To make the topping, combine all the ingredients in a separate dish and stir thoroughly.
- Then, evenly distribute the topping across the filling mix after placing it in the baking dish that has been previously prepared.
- The top should be golden brown after 20 minutes of baking.
- Serve hot.

6. CHOCOLATE CRUNCH BARS

 5 minutes 3 minutes 4 servings

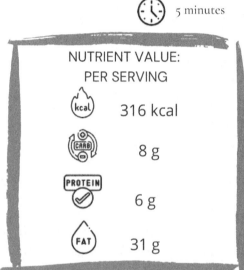

NUTRIENT VALUE:
PER SERVING

316 kcal

8 g

6 g

31 g

Ingredients

- ½ cups sugar-free chocolate chips
- 1 cup almond butter
- Stevia to taste
- ¼ cup coconut oil
- 3 cups pecans

Directions:

- Organize parchment paper in layers in an 8-inch baking pan.
- In a bowl, combine butter, coconut oil, as well as sweetener with chocolate chips.
- Microwave it for two to three minutes, stirring halfway through, to completely melt it.
- Add nuts and seeds and stir. Mix slowly.
- Spread this mixture evenly after pouring it into the baking pan.
- For two to three hours, refrigerate.
- Slice, then dish.

7. HOMEMADE PROTEIN BAR

 5 minutes 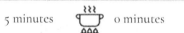 0 minutes 4 servings

Ingredients

- 1 cup nut butter
- Stevia, to taste
- ½ tsp. sea salt

- 4 tbsp. coconut oil
- 1 tsp. cinnamon (Optional)
- 2 scoops vanilla protein

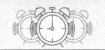

NUTRIENT VALUE:
PER SERVING

 179 kcal

 5 g

 6 g

14 g

Directions:
- Mix coconut oil with butter, protein, stevia, and salt in a dish.
- Stir in cinnamon and chocolate chip.
- Press the mixture firmly and freeze until firm.
- Cut the crust into small bars.
- Serve and enjoy.

8. SHORTBREAD COOKIES

 10 minutes   15 minutes   6 servings

NUTRIENT VALUE:
PER SERVING

288 kcal

10 g

8 g

14 g

Ingredients
- 2½ cups almond flour
- 6 tbsps. nut butter
- ½ cup erythritol
- 1 tsp. vanilla essence

Directions:
- Set the oven to 350 °F.
- Stack parchment paper on a cookie sheet.
- Beat butter with erythritol until fluffy.
- Stir in vanilla essence and almond flour. Mix well until becomes crumbly.
- Spoon out a tablespoon of cookie dough onto the cookie sheet.
- Add more dough to make as many cookies.
- Bake for 15 minutes until brown.
- Serve.

9. PEANUT BUTTER BARS

 10 minutes   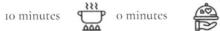 0 minutes   6 servings

Ingredients
- ¾ cup almond flour
- 2 oz. almond butter
- ¼ cup Swerve
- ½ cup peanut butter
- ½ tsp. vanilla

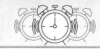
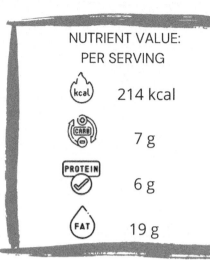

NUTRIENT VALUE:
PER SERVING

 214 kcal

7 g

 6 g

19 g

Directions:
- Combine all the ingredients for the bars.
- Transfer this mixture to a 6-inch small pan. Press it firmly.
- Refrigerate for 30 minutes.
- Slice and serve.

10. ZUCCHINI BREAD PANCAKES

🕐 15 minutes   🍲 8 minutes   🍽 3 servings

NUTRIENT VALUE:
PER SERVING

246 kcal

49 g

8 g

4 g

Ingredients
- 1 tbsp. grapeseed oil
- ½ cup chopped walnuts
- 2 cups walnut milk
- 1 cup shredded zucchini
- ¼ cup mashed burro banana
- 2 tbsps. date sugar
- 2 cup Kamut flour or spelled

Directions:

- Place the date sugar and flour into a bowl. Whisk together.
- Add in the mashed banana and walnut milk. Stir until combined. Remember to scrape the bowl to get all the dry mixture. Add in walnuts and zucchini. Stir well until combined.
- Place the grapeseed oil onto a griddle and warm.
- On the heated griddle, pour 1/4 cup of the batter. Leave it alone till surface bubbles start to appear. The pancake should be cooked through after four minutes of careful flipping.
- On the heated griddle, pour 1/4 cup of the batter.
- Leave it alone till surface bubbles start to appear. The pancake should be cooked through after four minutes of careful flipping.
- Place the pancakes onto a serving plate and enjoy with some agave syrup.

11. QUINOA PORRIDGE

 5 minutes   15 minutes   4 servings

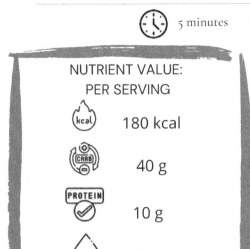

NUTRIENT VALUE:
PER SERVING

180 kcal

40 g

10 g

7 g

Ingredients

- Zest 1 lime
- ½ cup coconut milk
- ½ tsp. cloves
- 1½ tsp. ground ginger
- 2 cups spring water
- 1 cup quinoa
- 1 grated apple

Directions:

- Cook the quinoa according to the instructions on the package. When the quinoa has been cooked, drain well. Put it back into the pot and stir in spices.
- Add coconut milk and stir well to combine.
- Grate the apple now and stir well.
- Divide equally into bowls and add the lime zest on top. Sprinkle with nuts and seeds of choice.

12. APPLE QUINOA

 15 minutes 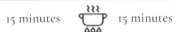 15 minutes 4 servings

Ingredients

- 1 tbsp. coconut oil
- Ginger
- ½ key lime
- 1 apple
- ½ cup quinoa

Optional Toppings

- Seeds
- Nuts
- Berries

NUTRIENT VALUE:
PER SERVING

 146 kcal

 16 g

 2 g

 9 g

Directions:

- Fix the quinoa according to the instructions on the package. When you are getting close to the end of the cooking time, grate the apple and cook for 30 seconds.
- Zest the lime into the quinoa and squeeze the juice in. Stir in the coconut oil.
- Divide evenly into bowls and sprinkle with some ginger.
- You can add in some berries, nuts, and seeds right before you eat.

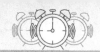
13. KAMUT PORRIDGE

 10 minutes 25 minutes 4 servings

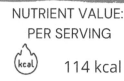

NUTRIENT VALUE:
PER SERVING

 114 kcal

24 g

 5 g

 10 g

Ingredients

- 1 cup kamut berries
- 1 tbsp. coconut oil
- ½ tsp. sea salt
- 4 tbsps. agave syrup
- 1 cup coconut milk

Optional Toppings

- Berries
- Coconut chips
- Ground nutmeg
- Ground cloves

Directions:

- You need to "crack" the Kamut berries. You can do this by placing the berries into a food processor and pulsing until you have 1¼ cups of Kamut.
- Put the cracked Kamut, salt, and coconut milk in a saucepan. Stir everything thoroughly to mix it. After allowing the mixture to fully boil, reduce the heat until the liquid is simmering. Once the Kamut becomes thicker to your preference, stir occasionally. Normally, this takes ten minutes.
- Take off the heat, stir in agave syrup and coconut oil.
- Garnish with toppings of choice and enjoy.

14. OVERNIGHT "OATS"

 5 minutes 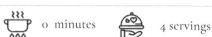 0 minutes 4 servings

Ingredients

- ½ cup berries
- ½ burro banana
- ½ tsp. ginger
- ½ cup coconut milk
- ½ cup hemp seeds

NUTRIENT VALUE:
PER SERVING

 139 kcal

 10 g

 9 g

 8 g

Directions:

- Put the hemp seeds, salt, and coconut milk into a glass jar. Mix well.
- Place the lid on the jar and put it in the refrigerator to sit overnight.
- The next morning, add the ginger, berries, and banana. Stir well and enjoy.

RECIPES SMOOTHIE & BEVERAGE

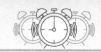
1. BERRY PROTEIN SMOOTHIE RECIPE

 5 minutes   0 minutes   6 servings

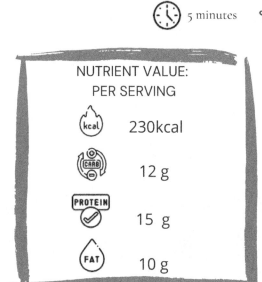

NUTRIENT VALUE:
PER SERVING

kcal   230kcal

CARB   12 g

PROTEIN   15 g

FAT   10 g

Ingredients

- 15.9 oz Strawberries (hulled) (450 g)
- 15.9 oz Blueberries (450 g)
- 15.9 oz Raspberries (450 g)
- 9 scoops ancient nutrition multi-collagen protein powder
- 33.8 fl oz Coconut milk (1 L can)
- 3.4 fl oz Keto Simple Syrup (to taste) (100 ml)
- 0.5 fl oz Lemon juice (15 ml)

Directions

- Combine the hulled strawberries, blueberries, and raspberries in a large mixing bowl.
- Add the ancient nutrition multi-collagen protein powder to the bowl.
- Pour in the coconut milk and keto simple syrup.
- Drizzle the lemon juice over the mixture for a touch of tanginess.
- Gently stir all the ingredients together until well combined.
- Serve this delicious and nutritious berry collagen smoothie as a refreshing treat.

2. CINNAMON ROLL KETO SHAKE

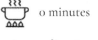 3 minutes   0 minutes   2 servings

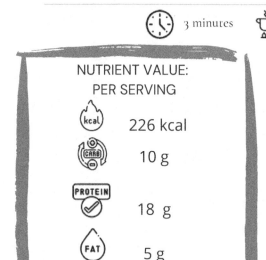

NUTRIENT VALUE:
PER SERVING

kcal   226 kcal

CARB   10 g

PROTEIN   18 g

FAT   5 g

Ingredients

- 7.4 fl oz milk or nut milk of choice (220 ml)
- 1 tsp vanilla extract (5 ml)
- 0.5 oz peanut butter powder (15 g)
- 1.1 oz cream cheese (30 g)
- 0.7 fl oz granulated erythritol (20 ml)
- 0.5 fl oz sugar-free maple syrup (15 ml)
- 0.4 oz ground cinnamon (10 g)
- 2 scoops bone broth protein powder
- 0.1 oz kosher salt (2 g)
- 8.8 oz ice (250 g)
- Whipped cream, ground cinnamon to garnish (optional)

Directions:

- Combine the milk or nut milk, vanilla extract, peanut butter powder, cream cheese, granulated erythritol, sugar-free maple syrup, ground cinnamon, bone broth protein powder, and kosher salt in a blender.
- Add the ice to the blender.
- Blend all the ingredients until smooth and well mixed.
- Pour the creamy mixture into the glasses.

- Optionally, add whipped cream and a pinch of ground cinnamon for extra flavor on top.
- Enjoy this delightful and nourishing protein-packed smoothie!

3. LUSCIOUS LIME SMOOTHIE

 10 minutes 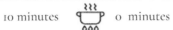 0 minutes 2 servings

NUTRIENT VALUE:
PER SERVING

 260 kcal

 9 g

 20 g

 2 g

Ingredients

- Juice of 2 limes
- 3-4 ice cubes
- 1 medium ripe avocado
- 2 tablespoons plain Greek yogurt (30 g)
- 1-2 tablespoons powdered erythritol or sweetener of choice
- 250 ml unsweetened coconut milk or almond milk
- Zest of 1 lime
- 1 scoop vanilla protein powder (optional)

Directions:

- Remove the pit by halving the ripe avocado. Place the meat in a blender by scooping.
- Pour in unsweetened coconut milk or almond milk.
- Squeeze the juice of 2 limes directly into the blender.
- Add the zest of 1 lime to enhance the citrus flavor.
- Spoon in the plain Greek yogurt for creaminess.
- Mix in one scoop of vanilla protein powder if you want more nutrition and taste.
- Sweeten the smoothie with powdered erythritol or your preferred sweetener. Adjust the sweetness to your liking.
- Drop in 3-4 ice cubes to chill the smoothie and make it refreshing.
- Blend all the ingredients until the mixture is smooth and velvety.
- Pour the luscious lime smoothie into a glass and enjoy the zesty and creamy goodness.

4. SHAMROCK SHAKE

 5 minutes 0 minutes 1 servings

NUTRIENT VALUE:
PER SERVING

 362 kcal

 5 g

 24 g

 0 g

Ingredients

- 2.6 oz vanilla protein powder of choice (75 g)
- 15.9 oz loosely packed spinach (450 g)
- 2.6 oz loosely packed fresh mint leaves (75 g)
- 4.2 oz mashed avocado or full-fat canned coconut milk (120 g)
- 8.5 fl oz nondairy milk of choice (250 ml)

Directions:

- Combine the vanilla protein powder, spinach, mint leaves, mashed avocado or coconut milk, and nondairy milk in a blender.
- Blend until all ingredients are well combined, and the mixture is smooth.

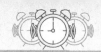

- If needed, you can adjust the consistency by adding more nondairy milk.
- Pour the smoothie into glasses and enjoy this nutritious and refreshing drink.
- This minty green protein smoothie is a great way to boost your protein intake while enjoying a burst of fresh flavors.

5. SUGAR-FREE CHOCOLATE SMOOTHIE

🕐 5 minutes   0 minutes   1 servings

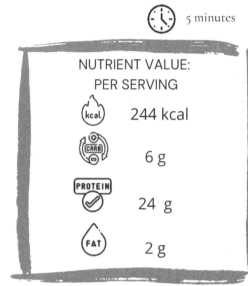

NUTRIENT VALUE:
PER SERVING

(kcal) 244 kcal

(CARB) 6 g

(PROTEIN) 24 g

(FAT) 2 g

Ingredients

- 2.5 fl oz unsweetened almond milk (75 ml)
- 1 oz Plain Greek yogurt (30 g)
- 0.35 oz no sugar added peanut butter (10 g)
- 0.07 fl oz vanilla extract (2 ml)
- 0.35 oz raw cacao powder or unsweetened cocoa powder (10 g)
- 1.1 oz collagen peptides (30 g)
- 3 ice cubes
- 1 pinch of sea salt
- optional: sugar-free sweetener to taste

Directions:

- Unsweetened almond milk, vanilla extract, Plain Greek yogurt, raw cacao or cocoa powder, ice cubes, collagen peptides, sugar-free peanut butter, and dash of sea salt should all be put in a blender.
- Unsweetened almond milk, vanilla extract, Plain Greek yogurt, raw cacao or cocoa powder, ice cubes, collagen peptides, sugar-free peanut butter, and a dash of sea salt should all be put in a blender.
- Blend until all ingredients are well mixed, and the smoothie is creamy.
- Please feel free to taste and add sugar-free sweetener if you'd like.
- Pour the smoothie into a glass and enjoy a nutritious and protein-packed treat.
- This delicious peanut butter chocolate smoothie is a great way to satisfy your cravings while nourishing your body with quality ingredients.

6. FAT BOMB SHAKE

🕐 5 minutes   0 minutes   1 servings

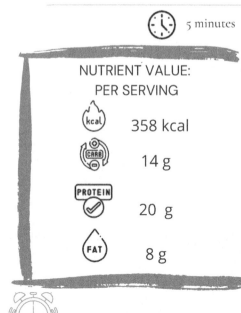

NUTRIENT VALUE:
PER SERVING

(kcal) 358 kcal

(CARB) 14 g

(PROTEIN) 20 g

(FAT) 8 g

Ingredients

- 3.5 oz frozen strawberries (100 g)
- 1 scoop vanilla protein powder
- Granulated or liquid stevia to taste (optional)
- 2.6 oz heavy cream (75 g)
- 1 cup unsweetened almond milk (250 ml)

Directions:

- Frozen strawberries, heavy cream, vanilla protein powder, and unsweetened almond milk should all be combined in a blender.
- Blend until the ingredients are well mixed, and the smoothie is creamy.

- Taste and add granulated or liquid stevia if you prefer a sweeter taste.
- Pour the smoothie into a glass and enjoy a delicious and refreshing treat packed with protein and flavor.
- This strawberry protein smoothie is a great way to start your day or refuel after a workout.

7. HEALTHY RED VELVET SMOOTHIE

 7 minutes 0 minutes 1 servings

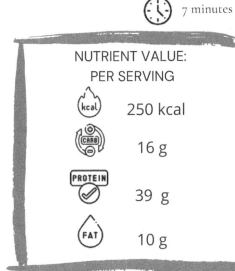

NUTRIENT VALUE:
PER SERVING

kcal 250 kcal

CARB 16 g

PROTEIN 39 g

FAT 10 g

Ingredients

- 1 ½ cups Unsweetened Vanilla Almond Milk (270 ml)
- 4.2 oz Plain, Nonfat Greek Yogurt (120 g)
- 3.5 oz Roasted Beet Puree (100 g)
- 1.1 oz Chocolate Whey Protein Powder (30 g)
- 0.35 oz Unsweetened Dutch Processed Cocoa Powder (10 g)
- 4 packets of Natural Sweetener (stevia, Truvia, etc.)

Directions:

- Blend the Roasted Beet Puree, Plain non-fat Greek Yogurt, and Chocolate Whey Protein Powder with unsweetened Dutch Processed Cocoa Powder in a blender.
- To taste, add the Natural Sweetener packets.
- Blend the ingredients until the smoothie is creamy and well-mixed.
- Pour the smoothie into a glass and enjoy a nutritious and flavorful beet-infused chocolate protein smoothie.
- This smoothie is a great way to incorporate beets and protein into your diet, and it makes for a satisfying and delicious snack or meal replacement.

8. MEAL REPLACEMENT SHAKE

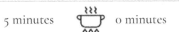 5 minutes 0 minutes 4 servings

NUTRIENT VALUE:
PER SERVING

 kcal 453 kcal

 CARB 6 g

 PROTEIN 8 g

 FAT 2 g

Ingredients

- 1 cup unsweetened almond milk (250 g)
- 1 medium avocado
- 2 tablespoons almond butter (30 g)
- 1/2 teaspoon cinnamon (2 g)
- 0.4 oz liquid stevia, or to taste (2 ml)
- 1/2 cup heavy cream (120 g)
- 2 tablespoons cocoa powder (30 g)
- 0.2 oz vanilla extract (1 g)
- 0.04 oz salt (1 g)
- 2 tablespoons golden flaxseed meal (30 g)
- 8 whole ice cubes

Directions:

- Heavy cream, along with almond milk should be blended together.
- The medium avocado, almond butter, flaxseed meal, cinnamon, liquid stevia, vanilla extract, as

well as salt should all be added.

- Toss in the ice cubes to chill and thicken the smoothie.
- Blend all the ingredients until the smoothie is creamy and well-mixed.
- Pour the smoothie into a glass and enjoy a rich and satisfying avocado-chocolate smoothie packed with healthy fats and nutrients.
- This smoothie is a delicious way to indulge while nourishing your body with wholesome ingredients.

9. COFFEE PROTEIN SMOOTHIE

 5 minutes 0 minutes   1 servings

NUTRIENT VALUE:
PER SERVING

 193 kcal

 19 g

 25 g

 9 g

Ingredients
- A few drops of stevia extract (1 ml)
- 1/2 cup vanilla almond milk (120 ml)
- Sprinkle cacao nibs, for topping if desired
- 1/2 cup brewed coffee (120 g)
- 1 ripe banana
- 2 cups cubed ice (300 g)
- 1 scoop of vanilla protein powder supplement (no sugar added)

Directions:
- Put the vanilla almond milk, banana, vanilla protein powder, then freshly brewed coffee in a blender.
- Add the cubed ice to the blender to chill and thicken the smoothie.
- If desired, add a few drops of stevia extract for extra sweetness.
- Blend all the ingredients until the smoothie is creamy and well-mixed.
- Please go ahead and pour the coffee banana smoothie into a glass and, if you'd like, sprinkle with cacao nibs for added texture and flavor.
- Enjoy a delightful and energizing blend of coffee and banana, perfect for a refreshing pick-me-up any day.

10. BEST DIET SHAKE

 5 minutes 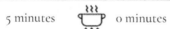 0 minutes 1 servings

Ingredients

- 2 tablespoons whipped cream, optional (30 g)
- 1 tablespoon Perfect Keto Nut Butter or almond butter (5 g)
- 2 tablespoons cacao powder (20 g)
- 1 ½ cup unsweetened oat milk (270 ml)
- 1/4 cup unsweetened coconut yogurt (60 ml)
- 1 ½ scoop of chocolate-flavored protein powder
- A few drops of liquid stevia, to taste (2 ml)

- 3–4 ice cubes
- 2 tablespoons cacao nibs, optional (10 g)

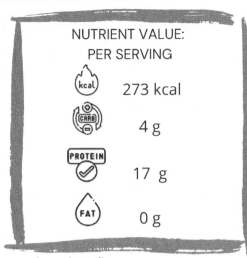

NUTRIENT VALUE:
PER SERVING

kcal — 273 kcal

CARB — 4 g

PROTEIN — 17 g

FAT — 0 g

Directions:

- Beat the full-fat coconut milk, chocolate whey protein powder unsweetened almond milk, and cacao powder together in a blender.
- To reach the correct degree of sweetness, add liquid stevia.
- Drop a tablespoon of Nut Butter or almond butter for a rich, nutty flavor.
- Toss in a few ice cubes to chill and thicken the smoothie.
- Blend all the ingredients until the mixture is smooth and well combined.
- Add cacao nibs for extra crunch and a burst of chocolate flavor.
- For an indulgent touch, top the smoothie with whipped cream.
- Pour into a glass and savor the delicious chocolate and nutty goodness blend.
- This smoothie is a satisfying and keto-friendly treat that you can enjoy guilt-free.

Scan the QR codes and get the Extra content designed for you!

SCAN ME DETOX

MONTHLY MEAL PLAN

DAYS	WEEK 1	WEEK 2	WEEK 3	WEEK 4
1	THE BUDDHA BOWL KETO MUSHROOM PASTA HALIBUT BLACKENED	FRITTATA WITH FETA CAULIFLOWER CURRY SOUP POT ROAST WITH FLAVOR	FLORENTINE EGG CASSEROLE KETO LASAGNA TUNA SALAD	THE FRENCH OMELET TARRAGON SALAD BAKED TURKEY
2	MIX TRAIL NOODLES WITH ZUCCHINI CITRUS SALMON	OMELET SOUTHWESTERN BLUE CHEESE ZOODLES CAULI SOUP	BOWL OF SAVORY OATS SALAD WITH CRISPY SPINACH CHICKEN SOUP	SCRAMBLED EGGS BREAKFAST BEEF TACO SOUP QUICK SALMON PATTIES
3	QUICHE CUPS WITH BROCCOLI KETO FETA BAKED PASTA MEAT TACOS	PANCAKES WITH KETO COCONUT FLOUR CREAMY TOMATO SOUP SALAD WITH ARUGULA	ALMOND FLOUR MUFFINS PESTO ZUCCHINI PASTA CHILI COD	FRITTATA WITH BACON & ASPARAGUS PASTA WITH CREAMY SALMON HEART OF ROMAINE GRILLED
4	FRITTATA WITH BACON & ASPARAGUS PASTA WITH CREAMY SALMON HEART OF ROMAINE GRILLED	LOW-CARB ENGLISH BREAKFAST LASAGNA WITH ZUCCHINI ROASTED BEEF WITH GRAVY	CRAB AVOCADO BOATS WILD MUSHROOM SOUP FILLETS OF HERB-ROASTED SALMON	STACK MASCARPONE-MUSHROOM FRITTATA CHICKEN TURNIP SOUP SALMON OVEN-ROASTED
5	SCRAMBLED SPINACH-MUSHROOM EGGS SALAD WITH CHICKEN AND ASPARAGUS ZUCCHINI CREAM SOUP	BREAKFAST CASSEROLE & GREEK FLAVORS CREAMY KETO PUMPKIN ALFREDO RUBBED TURKEY TS	SMOKED SALMON BREAKFAST SANDWICH PASTA CREAMY PESTO RUTABAGA THAI COCONUT SOUP	THE BUDDHA BOWL BACON-WRAPS CHICKPEA BOOSTER BOWL
6	BAKED APPLES FILLETS OF SEASONED TILAPIA SALAD WATERMELON & ARUGULA	OMELET SOUTHWESTERN SHRIMP ROASTED IN GARLIC ZUCCHINI PASTA GARLICKY CHICKEN SOUP	FRITTATA WITH FETA BUTTERNUT SQUASH RISOTTO KABOBS OF GINGER-TUNA	OMELET SOUTHWESTERN SALAD WITH A MINTY DRESSING FROM GREECE SMOTHERED TURKEY
7	QUINOA PORRIDGE PROVOLONE TURKEY CHEESE CREAMY BROCCOLI AND LEEK SOUP	APPLE QUINOA MEATBALLS WITH KETO SAUCE CREAMY BROCCOLI & CAULIFLOWER SOUP	THE FRENCH OMELET SALAD WITH CHICKEN AND ASPARAGUS WILD MUSHROOM SOUP	BERRY PROTEIN SMOOTHIE RECIPE SLOW-COOKER TURKEY WITH HERBS PARSLEY TUNA BOWLS

CONCLUSION

Congratulations! You've now journeyed through the fascinating world of intermittent fasting, uncovering its transformative power and potential for a healthier, more balanced life. As we conclude this empowering expedition, I want to reflect on the incredible knowledge we've amassed and the impact it can have on our well-being.

Throughout this enriching experience, we've delved deep into the various facets of intermittent fasting. From understanding its historical roots to exploring its science, we've gained valuable insights into how this age-old practice can revolutionize our health. We've seen how fasting can catalyze weight loss, longevity, and mental clarity, among many other remarkable benefits.

In our pursuit of knowledge, we unveiled hormones' significant role, particularly for women, as they navigate the fasting journey. We've learned how hormonal fluctuations can influence our responses to fasting and how intermittent fasting can help regulate hormonal imbalances, empowering women in their unique needs.

Beyond the physical, we've acknowledged the profound mental and emotional impact of intermittent fasting. It can strengthen our resolve, cultivate mindfulness, and foster a newfound self-awareness. With each fasting cycle, we become more attuned to the intricacies of our bodies, rekindling the long-lost connection between our mind, soul, and nourishment.

As we honed our understanding of nourishment, we carefully curated our feeding windows, embracing nutrient-dense foods that fuel our bodies and minds. By choosing wisely and steering clear of processed temptations, we laid the foundation for sustained vitality and resilience.

In our pursuit of a vibrant life, we've harmonized the art of fasting with the joy of physical activity. We've witnessed the synergy of strength when intermittent fasting and exercise unite to elevate our endurance, enhance our performance, and sculpt our bodies into marvels of health.

As we stand at the precipice of our intermittent fasting journey, let us remember that this is not just a diet but a profound lifestyle choice. It's a celebration of nourishing our bodies with intention, cherishing the gift of every meal, and savoring the moments when we abstain. It's an homage to our ancestors who understood the innate wisdom of fasting and a testament to our modern quest for holistic wellness.

CONCLUSION

Embrace this journey with an open heart and an adventurous spirit, for it holds the potential to transform not only your body but your entire way of being. As the days pass and the fasting hours tick by, you'll find a sense of empowerment that knows no bounds, a resilience that surges through every cell, and a renewed zest for life that defies expectations.

Remember, you are not alone on this path. Thousands of others have walked it before you, leaving footprints of inspiration and success. Draw from their experiences, and listen to your inner voice—it knows what's best for you.

So, my fellow fasting enthusiast, I encourage you to embark on this journey wholeheartedly, embracing its challenges, savoring its triumphs, and basking in the radiant glow of transformation. As you adopt intermittent fasting as a way of life, may you find the balance, clarity, and joy that has eluded you.

With newfound vitality and a soul nourished in wisdom, you can move forward fearlessly, ready to unlock the boundless potential that awaits you. As you go on this extraordinary path, always remember that the power lies within you, and intermittent fasting is your guiding light toward a life of holistic well-being.

Bon voyage on this awe-inspiring adventure, and may your journey be filled with abundant blessings, unshakable strength, and the sweet taste of triumph.

Your companion in wellness,

Laure Leller

INDEX

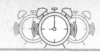

Made in the USA
Las Vegas, NV
17 April 2024